PRAISE FOR *Moving into Meditation*

"Gently humorous, deeply insightful, and always practical, Anne Cushman helps us go straight to the heart of our own basic goodness amid the messiness of our everyday lives. I can't wait to share Anne's insight with the women I teach. Her willingness to share her own life journey will give us all the confidence we need to come home to ourselves in a loving, nonjudgmental way."
—Linda Sparrowe, author of *The Woman's Book of Yoga and Health*

"With a light touch and her characteristic humor, Anne draws us into her own life story as she leads us into mindful exercises with simple clarity and kindness. There is never a dull sentence! In *Moving into Meditation* there is no rigidity or expectation—as is so often experienced in public classes—but rather the sense of time, space, freedom, and encouragement to explore your own needs. She is not offering a well-trodden path; she is drawing from her own life and practice, where yoga and meditation flow together into the same river of awareness. This is a book of valuable guidelines that will provide inspiration and encouragement to even the most seasoned practitioner of yoga and meditation."
—-Angela Farmer, yoga pioneer and creator of
The Feminine Unfolding, Inner Body Flow, and other videos

"Anne Cushman's *Moving into Meditation* is more than a book. It is an entire program for cultivating a mindful relationship with the body. In the Four Foundations of Mindfulness teaching, the Buddha says to begin with awareness of the body. Anne's book provides a pathway for establishing a body-based meditation practice that is in accordance with this instruction. Very specific and well organized, this book allows you to establish a mindful yoga practice at your own pace. For those who struggle with body challenges, it offers specific heart meditation practices to bring about change in how you relate to your body. The amount of detailed information in this book makes it a reference within itself."
—Phillip Moffitt, author of *Dancing with Life* and
Emotional Chaos to Clarity

"Anne Cushman's new book is a rich meal indeed. Cushman is one of the most talented writers in the contemplative world today. Her prose is elegant and engaging, vibrating with intelligent life force. But beyond that, she has digested the histories of the yoga and Buddhist traditions so fully that she is able to make a stunning and seamless integration of the two—and to give us an unparalleled explication of why, indeed, they are *not* two traditions but one. As if that were not enough, she weaves all of this together into a practical, useful, inspiring, accurate, and comprehensive twelve-week program of study and practice. Wow! This book should soon be on the shelf of every meditator and yogi who aspires to a full embrace of practice and of life."
—Stephen Cope, author of *Yoga and the Quest for the True Self*

Moving *into* Meditation

A 12-Week
Mindfulness Program
for Yoga Practitioners

Anne Cushman

 Shambhala *Boston & London* 2014

Shambhala Publications, Inc.
Horticultural Hall
300 Massachusetts Avenue
Boston, Massachusetts 02115
www.shambhala.com

9 8 7 6 5 4 3 2 1

First Edition
Printed in the United States of America

♾ This edition is printed on acid-free paper that meets the
American National Standards Institute Z39.48 Standard.
♻ This book is printed on 30% postconsumer recycled paper.
For more information please visit www.shambhala.com.

Distributed in the United States by Penguin Random House LLC
and in Canada by Random House of Canada Ltd

Designed by James D. Skatges

Library of Congress Cataloging-in-Publication Data

Cushman, Anne, author.
Moving into meditation: a 12-week mindfulness program
for yoga practitioners / Anne Cushman.—First edition.
Pages   cm
ISBN 978-1-61180-098-2 (paperback)
1. Meditation—Buddhism. 2. Yoga. I. Title.
BQ5612.C88 2014
294.3'4436—dc23
2013042189

Contents

Prologue

Here's the one thing I know for sure about moving into meditation: The only time you can do it is now.

I mean, right now. Even if you haven't answered your e-mail or paid the IRS or thrown out the three-week-old pasta that's festering at the back of your fridge or fixed the broken screen door that's banging in the rising wind of an incoming storm. Even if the person you're in love with just fell in love with someone else. Even if your kids have commandeered all of your meditation cushions and yoga mats to build an obstacle course in your living room.

Glaciers are melting, hurricanes pound one coast while wildfires rage down the other, and you are behind on three deadlines on a job you know you're lucky to have. People you love have died. And you're beginning to suspect that someday you might too.

So what you are going to do, in the midst of all of this, is stop. Sense the soles of your feet, the tender palms of your hands. Hear the chirping of the wrens or the rumble of the garbage truck. Smell the eucalyptus trees, the cat litter, the antiseptic in the hospital halls, the faint whiff of cinnamon scones wafting from the corner bakery. Gaze up at what you can see of the infinite sky, even if it's just a chip of blue in the corner of your window—even if you have to close your eyes to imagine it waiting for you, somewhere outside the box of concrete and wood and steel you're packed inside. Feel your fragile, astonishing human body, your weird and magnificent human life.

Introduction

In the winter of 1999—when I'd been practicing both yoga and Buddhist meditation for about a decade and a half—I started teaching yoga on retreats at Spirit Rock Meditation Center, a Buddhist oasis nestled in the golden, rolling hills north of San Francisco.

The retreatants at Spirit Rock had not come there planning to learn yoga postures. (My computer's spell-checker wants me to call them "retreat ants," which strikes me as a wonderful metaphor for the diligence with which spiritual seekers tunnel into the depths of their lives while often hauling emotional loads bigger than their own bodies.) They were there to train with a cadre of Buddhist teachers in the art of mindfulness meditation—which, like most people, they generally thought of as something that was practiced while sitting still.

Some of them had come because their lives had been shredded—a brain tumor, a shattered marriage, the collapse of a business, the death of a best friend. Others were just looking for a sanctuary from the daily thunder of e-mails and traffic. When I first started teaching there, I was newly married and grieving a daughter who had died at birth. Over the coming years, I taught on retreats while pregnant, while nursing a baby, while divorcing, while raising a son.

In a sheltered valley shared with bobcats, deer, turkeys, lizards, and the occasional mountain lion, we would sit for hours in silence while winter rains drummed on the soaring roof of the meditation hall. We'd do walking meditation on paths winding through spring irises or sun-scorched summer hills—then pick ticks off our pant legs before returning to sit again.

In those days, yoga was not permitted in the main meditation hall—one meditation teacher joked that the Buddha seated cross-legged on the altar might be offended by the sight of so many buttocks uplifted in Downward Dog. The retreatants were more likely to be wearing baggy jeans or peasant skirts than stretchy leggings. So every day we went to a small upstairs room where I taught gentle but powerful movement, breath, and energy practices from the hatha yoga tradition. These brought relief to backs, necks, and shoulders knotted by hours of seated meditation. But more important, meditators reported that the yoga opened up a new way of connecting with the practice of mindful presence—and helped them embody their meditative awakenings as they moved back into the chaos and beauty of their daily lives.

And although I was there in the role of a teacher, what I mainly noticed was how much I was learning from the retreatants—their courage and vulnerability as they turned to face themselves again and again. What kind of practices should I offer people who came to the yoga sessions so sensitive and open, as if, in the shrine of silence, they'd removed the protective armor around their hearts? The writer Annie Dillard tells her students, "Write as if you are dying; or as if you are writing for an audience consisting solely of dying people. That is, after all, the case." How could I teach with that kind of depth?

Based on these explorations, in 2006 I began to codirect (with the Spirit Rock guiding teacher Phillip Moffitt) an eighteen-month program training yoga teachers to integrate mindfulness meditation into their practice. Unlike most meditators, the yoga teachers arrived at Spirit Rock wearing workout clothes and carrying rolled-up mats, foam blocks, and an arsenal of straps, bolsters, blankets, and eye pillows. But like anyone else, they were also carrying their lives, a bubbling stew of heartbreak and happiness. A mother was grieving two children killed in a fire. One couple got pregnant during the training and brought their nursing baby to the final ten-day retreat. Between sessions, gang violence left the home of a young woman trainee riddled with bullets.

Over the course of the training, they brought into their practice of yoga postures and breathing techniques the practices of meditation and heart-mind training that have always been part of the true yogi's path. And they explored the questions that yogis have been asking for centuries: How do we live with wisdom and compassion in these human bodies, these human hearts, these human minds and spirits? How do we find deep joy and meaning in a world where everything dear to us will eventually slip from our grasp?

These are the questions that *Moving into Meditation* is intended to explore. It's a systematic program designed for yoga practitioners of all levels who want to deepen their practice of physical postures and breathing techniques to support, express, and include the ancient art of mindfulness meditation. It's for people who want to attend not just to the body but also to the heart and mind, intentionally cultivating kind, moment-to-moment presence for every experience, from frying an egg or writing an e-mail to dancing at a wedding or sitting by the bedside of a dying friend.

First taught by the Buddha more than twenty-five hundred years ago, mindfulness meditation has recently exploded in popularity as scientists document a host of benefits that include reducing stress, boosting compassion, improving sleep, lowering risk of depression, slowing cellular aging, and even increasing gray matter in the brain. Over the course of this twelve-week program

- You'll learn how to practice yoga postures as meditation in motion, inviting you into a deeper intimacy with your body, breath, heart, and mind.
- You'll nourish your inner peace and stability through connecting with and freeing your breath.
- You'll cultivate a daily home practice of seated meditation that's solidly grounded in your felt sense of your body.
- And you'll progressively develop the ability to know more deeply and relate more wisely to every part of your inner and outer life—the sensations of body and breath, the ebb and flow of emotions, the twitter of thoughts, the unpredictable and ever-changing circumstances in which you find yourself.

▆ This isn't just a book—if you want, it can be a multimedia experience. If you'd like to get a taste right now of what it's like to move into meditation, just go to annecushman.com/practices and I'll lead you through some downloadable guided video practices, so you can experience for yourself how powerful mindful yoga can be.

Throughout this book, practices marked with a ◀») include links to downloadable audio. Practices marked with a ◼ include links to downloadable video.

Almost everywhere these days, you can find excellent yoga classes where you can learn the basics of yoga alignment and be guided through a sequence of postures that will improve your strength and flexibility, reduce your stress, and increase your joy. But the vast majority of classes include little or no instruction in the art of seated meditation, even though meditation is fundamental to the classical yoga tradition.

You can also find many wonderful courses and retreats where you can learn the practice of mindfulness meditation. However, most of those offerings do not explicitly build on the skill and sensitivity to body, breath, and energy that you are developing in your yoga practice.

This twelve-week program is your chance to explore and integrate yoga and mindfulness meditation in a unified way, within the cauldron of your own individualized home practice. It's not an instruction manual of yoga postures (of which there are many excellent ones available)—in fact, the program assumes that you are already familiar with the yoga basics. Rather, it's designed to help you learn how to use these physical forms as a vehicle for becoming more intimate with yourself and your world. Rather than specific asanas, it teaches *ways of paying attention* that can illuminate and transform your practice whether you're a relative beginner or a seasoned practitioner.

Over twelve weeks you'll use the forms of asana, pranayama (breath cultivation), and meditation to progressively deepen your connection with and understanding of your body, heart, and mind—not the perfect body, heart, and mind that you might achieve sometime in the distant future through a raw vegan diet, daily workouts, and decades of psychotherapy but the flawed and miraculous ones you already inhabit. The forms of yoga will become a gateway to the practice of fundamental principles that can help you live a sensitive, responsive, and embodied life.

WHY PRACTICE MINDFUL YOGA?

These days, most people who hear the word *yoga* think of an activity that's primarily physical: a lithe young woman bending, leaping, and sweating through a stress-busting, butt-lifting workout. And when they hear the word *meditation,* they think of an activity that's primarily mental: a black-robed Zen monk with a shaved head sitting cross-legged on a cushion.

But as you know if you've ever set your bare feet on a yoga mat, the first thing that happens when you start to explore your body is that you slam into your mind. Flow through a series of yoga poses, and if you're paying attention, you'll see the full range of human emotion flowing along with you—joy, frustration, envy, bliss, self-loathing. Fold into a forward bend and the frozen sorrow in your lower back melts into a river of tears. A back bend cracks open the sealed chamber of terror behind your heart.

And sit down on a meditation cushion, and there is your body—perhaps a teeny bit angry that you've been keeping it waiting for so long. That aching back, those throbbing knees, that knife between the shoulders you've been pretending wasn't there. That wave of bliss that starts at the base of your spine and ripples up with every breath—but melts away as soon as you try to grasp it. Drop beneath your racing thoughts and find your clenched jaw. Step into a tornado of terror and feel your belly churning.

Yogi is the ancient Sanskrit name for anyone who ventures into this territory of conscious inner sensing and investigation. And what yogis discover, again and again, is that mind and body and heart are not separate, solid entities. They are different aspects of an interpenetrating continuum of experience, fluidly changing breath by breath, moment by moment.

As a yogi, you need a practice that deliberately integrates the physical, mental, and emotional aspects of your being. You need an asana practice that opens you to the currents of your heart and mind. You need a meditation practice that is grounded in a sensuous connection with your body.

The word *yoga,* of course, has never just meant physical postures. It's an umbrella term that encompasses a wide range of intertwined psychological, spiritual, and physical practices and traditions with their roots in the fertile spiritual soil of ancient India—including both the meditation practices taught by the Buddha and the physical practices most people commonly associate with yoga today.

The naked ascetic with matted dreadlocks smoking ganja by the banks of the Ganges, his body covered with ash from a funeral pyre— he's doing yoga. The old woman in the Shiva temple, chanting Sanskrit prayers and scattering flower petals in front of a polished stone lingam dripping with ghee—she's doing yoga too. So is the volunteer at the ashram soup kitchen ladling out stew to homeless people.

In its oldest form, the word *yoga* comes from the ancient Sanskrit verb *yuj*, which is a cognate of our English word *yoke*. And like the word *yoke*, *yoga* connotes both discipline and connection. Yoga is the discipline of creating connection—or, more accurately, revealing the deep connection that is already there. It's about connecting with your own beautiful, breaking-down body, your own vast and vulnerable heart; with the redwood tree tapping at your window and the woman with broken teeth by the freeway on-ramp holding a sign that says "will work for food."

This quality of present-moment connection is also implicit in the Buddhist term *mindfulness*. "Mindfulness" is one English translation of the Pali word *sati*, which is also sometimes translated as "awareness" or more literally "remembering." It's our innate capacity to remember that we are right here in the moment: awake to our laughter, to a honking horn, to the smell of a lemon. It's the quality of our heart and mind that knows what is happening right now—without judging it, pushing it away, or trying to hang on to it.

In a sense, then, the term *mindful yoga* is redundant. If it isn't mindful, it isn't really yoga at all. Yoga *is* this state of intimate, unentangled presence—and it's also the tools of body, breath, heart, and mind that we use to cultivate it.

It's vital for contemporary hatha yoga practitioners to have a way of going deeper into the meditative aspects of their practice. Yoga asanas and pranayama are designed to open the body and the energy systems: At the end of a well-sequenced yoga session, your nervous system is calm and balanced and your mind is relaxed and energized. You have a steady inner platform on which to sit in meditation and look a little deeper into your true nature. You're beautifully prepared to drink deeply from the pool of inner stillness and to investigate the patterns of habitual thinking that keep you from diving even deeper.

Yet what most people do instead is get off their mat, put on their shoes, hop in their cars or onto the subways, and head out for the rest of their day.

And sadly, while most contemporary yoga classes pay lip service to the ideals of mindfulness and meditative presence, often the style in which they are taught is not conducive to cultivating those qualities. You can spend years polishing advanced yoga postures without acquiring the skills you actually need to help you navigate the rough seas of life. How does your yoga practice help you when your best friend dies in a car crash? When your teenager gets hooked on drugs? When a factory is dumping chemicals into the river from which your community gets its drinking water?

However, without the tools of a yogic embodiment art, you can also spend years as a meditator locked in the small, dark closet of your own mind—endlessly battling inner demons without learning how to work with your body and nervous system to cultivate the inner environment in which peace, compassion, and ease can naturally flourish.

The good news is that it's fairly easy to get these practices to work together. You can enrich your asana practice by seasoning it with mindfulness; you can enrich your meditation practice by grounding it in your body. Together, these practices can generate a quality of connected, intimate presence. Not a mindfulness like a hothouse orchid that can thrive only in rarified, retreat settings but a hardy weed like dandelions or clover that you can't dig out of your lawn no matter how hard you try. And once this quality of presence is firmly rooted, you can use it to investigate and loosen ingrained patterns of thought and action that may be keeping you trapped.

WHAT IS MINDFUL YOGA?

When I mention that I teach yoga on meditation retreats, the first question I get is always, "What kind of yoga do you teach?"

I usually answer something like, "I teach yoga as a support for and expression of meditative presence and awakening."

There is a pause, and then my interrogator generally asks again, with a hint of an exasperated sigh: "Yes, but what *kind* of yoga?"

The fact is, all of the different flavors of yoga that make up the menu of many yoga studios—Iyengar, Ashtanga, Viniyoga, Anusara, Bikram, Kripalu, yin, and an ever-multiplying array of other brand names—are simply modern combinations and brandings of various elements of the yogic tool kit. These various types of yoga may emphasize different aspects of and approaches to the practice. But all of them are variations of hatha yoga—the art of transforming consciousness by working directly with the physical form. And they all share a common goal—enlivening the physical body while liberating the heart and mind.

Because of this, any "style" of yoga can be practiced as a support for and expression of mindfulness meditation. (And any style, of course, can also be practiced as a mindless workout. It's your choice.) One is not better than another. Different paths are appropriate for different people at different times—and choosing the approach that's right for your unique body is a mindfulness practice in itself. What works for a teenage gymnast won't be the right practice for a woman who's eight months' pregnant or a middle-aged accountant who sits at a desk all day or a professional weight lifter or an elder in a wheelchair.

When you're practicing mindful yoga, your emphasis is not on *what* you're doing but on *how* you're doing it. You're practicing in a way that is intimately in touch with your body, your breath, your heart, and your mind. You're using the forms of stillness and movement to feel into a spaciousness that lies beyond both. The idea is not to cram your practice into a new form called "mindful" yoga. The idea is to liberate it into a deeper expression of and support for your inner journey.

For that reason, I focus less on specific poses and more on practices, principles, reflections, and suggestions that can help you take your own yoga even deeper, whatever your unique path may be. These are principles that can be practiced whether you are a beginner to yoga asana or an advanced practitioner—whether you are fit and strong or you are ill or injured or have limited mobility. And whatever forms you use to explore these principles, what you will spiral back into is the reality of your own unfolding life.

HOW TO USE THIS BOOK

While long periods of silent retreat are wonderful, most of us don't spend our lives in this mode—and even those who can go on retreats generally have to return to a busy life between them. So this book is designed to help you investigate in a systematic way the practices and teachings that you might delve into in a yoga and meditation retreat—while continuing your normal activities of going to meetings, falling in love, sautéing broccoli, and posting status updates online.

Its week-by-week format encourages you to take the time to investigate each aspect of the practice with some depth so it has a chance to take root in your body and nervous system, becoming an integrated part of who you are. I've offered some of the practices that I've found most helpful—both in my own practice and in my students'—in taking "mindful yoga" from a concept to a lived reality. Throughout the book, audio ◀» and video ◾ practices help you deepen your exploration still further.

Over the course of the program, you'll systematically build your embodied understanding of mindfulness practice. In weeks 1 and 2 we'll focus on mindfulness of the physical body in stillness and in motion. In weeks 3 and 4 we'll turn our attention to getting to know our breath. We'll dive more deeply into seated meditation in week 5; and in week 6 we'll turn our attention to standing and walking meditation.

In week 7 we'll focus on using our practice to encourage and embody an open heart toward ourselves and others. Weeks 8 through 10 will develop our awareness of our emotions and thoughts, and in week 11 we'll examine how to work with some of the common obstacles to clarity. Finally, in week 12 we'll use the presence and sensitivity that we've cultivated to look more deeply at the nature of our selves and our world.

Dividing up the practice in this way is, of course, somewhat artificial. Practice is an ever-deepening and never-ending spiral, and twelve weeks just scratches the surface of what will be a lifetime journey. And in reality, all of the aspects of the practice intermingle to form one organic whole. How can you explore your body without also sensing your breath? How can you feel your breath without also tasting the emotions that saturate each one? That's a bit like saying, "Look at that red horse—but don't look at the red part, just the horse part." But inviting a particular dimension of our experience into the foreground for a while can help us cultivate a new kind of intimacy with it, like having a deep conversation with a single person in the midst of a crowded party. And by the end of the twelve weeks—to strain the metaphor a bit—you'll be able to dance with everyone there.

I've deliberately made this book personal—exploring and revealing my own life journey as I encourage you to explore your own. I've also included stories and insights from other dedicated practitioners of mindful yoga and meditation, most of them graduates of the training I lead at Spirit Rock and many of them now teaching mindful yoga themselves.

I've included these stories because compassionate mindful presence does not occur in a void; it's planted and grows in the fertile meadows and rocky crags of our wild journeys. And ultimately, all of these practices and themes are just intended to point us back to the connection with the bones and blood of our lives: the roar of the freeway traffic, the smell of the salt wind off the ocean, the tender spot we kiss on the top of a baby's head, our tears as we scatter a loved one's ashes.

PART ONE ✎ Foundations

CHAPTER 1

My Journey into Mindful Yoga

WHEN I WALKED into my very first yoga class back in 1980, if you had told me that someday I would be teaching mindfulness meditation to yoga practitioners, I would have thought that you were out of your mind. It was my freshman year at a high-powered East Coast university, and I was a brainy, disheveled bookworm with ambitions to be a journalist—I had signed up for yoga only to satisfy the PE requirement. The class was taught by a turbaned kundalini teacher with a Texas accent and an Indian name that had been given to him by his Sikh guru. At our first session he informed us that he was going to go around the room and check each student to make sure our chakras were spinning properly. As he got closer and closer, I got more and more nervous. I had chakra performance anxiety: I was sure that when he examined me, he would shake his head gravely and say, "I've never seen anything like it. You don't have any chakras at all!" In a panic, I ducked out and hid in the women's bathroom until I was sure that part of the class was over.

A few weeks later the yoga sessions ended abruptly when he eloped with one of my fellow undergraduates—someone, I presumed, with really magnificent chakras. With a combination of relief and regret, I fulfilled my PE requirement by signing up for tennis.

However, my interest in Eastern philosophies and practices continued to grow. In my junior year I became a religion major with a focus on Buddhism and Hinduism. I hoped that my studies would illuminate more about those mysterious chakras. Mainly, though, they entailed huddling in my basement library carrel, drinking bad coffee from a vending machine under the flickering greenish glow of fluorescent lights, and poring over mountains of texts that told me that what I was looking for couldn't be found in books. So the summer between my junior and senior years, at the recommendation of one of my professors, I flew out to a Zen center in Southern California to spend a month doing field research.

The Zen center was just off Wilshire Boulevard in south Los Angeles; at night I could hear the crackle of gunfire in the neighborhood. I arrived there wearing a pink embroidered shirt and a white flounced hippie skirt, which I only belatedly realized was not standard monastic attire. Before I could meet the Japanese *roshi*—Zen master—I was told to spend a day in a room alone, sitting cross-legged on an understuffed black cushion facing a blank white wall. I was not to get off my meditation cushion except to use the bathroom. (I found myself peeing frequently as a source of entertainment.) At lunchtime a plate of brown rice and broccoli was left outside my door. I was given no other instructions other than to "watch my breath."

My knees hurt. My back hurt. I was restless and bored. I had expected meditating to be blissful, like a trip on some new kind of drug. But instead, the thing it most reminded me of was racing cross-country in high school—pounding on for mile after mile through forests of crimson autumn maples, side cramping, breath catching, at the limits of my physical and mental endurance, with some squealing, feeble part of my mind scheming for ways to get out of the race without losing face: *I could pretend to twist my ankle . . . I could fake a heart attack. . . .*

I spent a month at the Zen center learning the seated meditation practice known as *zazen,* which was described to me as a formal practice for cultivating an awake, relaxed alertness you could then bring to your whole life. As part of my daily practice, I chopped vegetables and raked the gravel pathways that wound around the carp pond. Many of the residents were monks—primarily Westerners, both men and women—with shaved heads, black robes, and luminous eyes. They struck me as peaceful and grounded, qualities I longed to experience for myself. But I had no idea how to get there.

In zazen instruction, my teachers paid a lot of attention to the physical details of the seated meditation posture—the upright seat, the crossed legs, the exact position of the hands in the mudra at the *hara,* or lower belly. Body awareness was implicit in the instructions I was given for work meditation: *Pay attention as you sweep the walk, wash the dishes, scrub a toilet. These activities are as much meditation as what you do on the cushion.* But what I would later come to know as the yogic embodiment arts—practices for cultivating the body to awaken the heart and mind—were not part of my Zen training.

Without this element, the moment-to-moment presence and ease that my Zen teacher spoke about—and that he and many of the senior practitioners radiated—remained an elusive concept for me. It was an ideal that I was striving for through my mind but could not find as a felt sense in my body.

After I graduated from college, I moved to New Mexico and found a home with two massage students in a wood-heated adobe cabin on the southern border of Santa Fe, out where the art galleries and million-dollar villas disintegrated into a tattered fringe of vacant lots and trailer parks. After digging her fingers into the university-induced knots in my upper back, one of my roommates invited me to an early-morning yoga class at the massage school. It was led by a slender man with muscles so clearly defined that the massage teacher regularly had him strip to his underwear to use him as an animated anatomy text. He stood at the front of the room in threadbare gray sweatpants, naked from the waist up. As he swung his arms overhead in a Sun Salutation, slabs of muscles slid around his chest and back; then he folded in two at the hips. I took a deep breath and dove in too.

And as I folded, arched, breathed, and sweated, I could feel that something different was starting to happen. My body thrummed like a plucked guitar string. Energy buzzed and tingled in my spine. I could feel my breath pulse through my whole body—rippling my vertebrae, spreading my ribs, sending waves of sensation through bones, muscles, organs, and skin.

Meditation, for me, had so far been a cerebral experience, with "me" sitting firmly in my own head, observing my breath and body (that itchy nostril! that stabbing knee!) like a theater critic reviewing a particularly maddening play. But now, for the first time, I was feeling my own body from the inside, swimming in a swirling stream of sensations. After years of trying to *watch* my breath, finally I was *being* it. In my meditation practice, I'd had my nose pressed to the glass of a shop window, peering in at a display of peace and happiness on the other side. With my yoga practice, the glass—even if only momentarily—was melting away.

From that moment onward, Buddhist meditation and hatha flowed together for me—not as separate practices but as two powerful currents of the same river. On vipassana retreats in California, I'd duck out of walking meditation to do Sun Salutations amid the pine trees and yuccas. On Zen retreats at Plum Village in France, I'd get up at dawn to stand on my head on the dewy grass outside my tent, while the sun rose over fields of sunflowers. As I sat in meditation, I'd feel the tingle and pulse of the energy I'd awakened through yoga postures. And at the heart of a sweaty yoga practice, I could rest in the stillness I'd cultivated while I sat on my cushion.

In the early days of my practice, taking a yoga break in the middle of a meditation retreat always felt a little illicit, as if I were sneaking out to have a margarita and get laid. Back then, most hard-core Buddhist practitioners looked down on yoga as excessively sensual and body obsessed—after all, how could you take seriously a spiritual practice that was performed in pink Lycra tights?

Meanwhile, in my yoga asana training, most of my teachers relegated seated meditation to a few minutes at the end of class, after emerging from the deep relaxation of Savasana. From the point of view of a handstanding, backflipping yoga athlete, Buddhist meditators were sedentary, out of shape, and shockingly out of touch with their bodies: they slumped on their beaten-down meditation cushions and tended to look lousy in leotards. Some teachers even warned that meditation was dangerous: if you sat still too long, you could go insane.

But I continued to combine the two traditions into one seamless practice. For me there was no faster way to transform my mind and heart than to move my body. Yoga offered me direct access to a joy that seemed to arise straight from my nerves and bones, independent of external circumstances. In Western terms, this transformation might be ascribed to hormones and nerve synapses and endorphins; in Eastern terms, to the life force energy of prana flowing through a network of subtle channels and vortexes. But in either case, my experience was the same—a transformation of all the subjective sensations that gave rise to my sense of self.

Moving my body into different shapes, I became a different person. Creating more space in my joints, I made more space in my mind as well. Twisting and bending and arching my body, I broke up the ice floes of self-judgment that had frozen in my muscles. I squeezed out the anxiety knotted between my shoulder blades. I melted the anger in the pit of my stomach into tears.

In the mid-1990s, I made a pilgrimage to India to visit the places associated with the Buddha's life. I explored the buried ruins of monasteries marking the site of his childhood palace. I hiked up a heat-baked hill to meditate in the tiny, smoke-blackened cave where he spent six years in ascetic practice. As lemur monkeys quarreled in the sal trees, I circumambulated a stupa commemorating the place where he died of food poisoning in his eighties.

My trip to India brought home for me a very simple truth: The Buddha was a human being, in a human body. Like any other person, he was born, walked on the earth, and died. And his great awakening took place in and through this body—a body that, like anyone else's, got sick, got hungry, shat, pissed, fell apart.

After all, I realized, most of the experiences that I thought of as most spiritual—being born, giving birth, loving another person, losing loved ones to death, facing death myself—were also intensely physical, inextricably entwined with the messy, sensual business of blood and nerves and skin.

An embodied practice grounded my awareness, again and again, in cartilage, muscle, organs, and bone. It reminded me that the specifics of my physical experience in any moment—this belly full of oatmeal, this pelvis skewed slightly to the right from years of carrying a baby on a hip, this sorrow shrink-wrapped around my heart—were the place where I touched the whole of creation. As I explored the wilderness of my own body, I saw that I was made of blood and bones, sunlight and water, pesticide residues and redwood humus, the fears and dreams of generations of ancestors.

When I started doing yoga, I actually thought there was somewhere to get to. Shuffling through old files recently, I found a yoga exam from my days in a teacher-training program at the Iyengar Yoga Institute in San Francisco in the late 1980s in which the teacher had asked us to pick four poses that we found difficult and describe what we were going to do to master them. Earnestly, I laid out my challenges—the tight hips in Revolved Triangle Pose, the tucked-under sitting bones in Seated Forward Bend—and outlined the steps I was taking to eradicate them. Implicit in my answer was the belief that my challenges were both finite and soluble, that with diligent practice I would root them out and arrive at perfection.

In those days I still thought that "doing things right" was the point of yoga. Through my practice, I imagined, I'd root out all of my messy imperfections: my tight hamstrings, my rambling mind, my possessiveness and jealousy, the way my left shoulder lifted higher than the right. Like my Downward Dog Pose, my whole life would come into perfect alignment. Nowadays my practice is different. My body has not gotten better and better, like an upgraded software program. Instead, despite my best efforts, it's wearing out, breaking down, growing softer and looser and weaker. My practice has gotten softer, kinder—focused less on *what* I'm practicing and more on *how*. These days I can't do the drop-back back bends I used to do effortlessly. When I stand on my head, my face slides down toward my hairline in a way I'm quite sure it didn't used to do. My practice is teaching me to embrace imperfection: to have compassion for all the ways things haven't turned out as I planned, in my body and in my life; for the way things keep falling apart and failing and breaking down. It's less about fixing things and more about learning to be present for exactly what is.

My practice has helped me be present through the terrible loss of delivering my stillborn daughter, Sierra, and the almost unbearable joy of receiving my newborn son, Skye, in my arms, wet and wide-eyed and lifting his wobbly head to turn toward his daddy's voice. It has helped me navigate divorce and midlife dating and raising a boy from diapers and bubble blowing to wilderness trips and Internet surfing. It's taught me to embrace my body and my life in all of their ragged edges and cellulite. It reminds me how futile are all of my attempts to control my body and my life and that when it comes right down to it, I can't control or hang on to anything that's really important.

But it also reminds me that despite all of this—or perhaps because of it—my life is precious and glorious. It's teaching me to find some sort of balance and ease in the uncertainty, as if I were doing a handstand poised at the edge of a cliff.

When I move into meditation these days, I feel like one of those yogis I used to see in India doing a headstand in the center of a circle of fire or sitting in lotus by a funeral pyre on the banks of the Ganges watching a corpse burn. I know the world is in flames all around me, I know my body is on its way back to the earth. But in the middle of it all, I can breathe and stretch and flow and dance; I can reach my arms to the sky and bow my head to the earth and feel my body ringing like a temple bell.

◼ To take your own guided journey through mindful yoga, go to annecushman.com/practices.

CHAPTER 2

Why Move into Meditation?

IN THE DECADES since I first began my spiritual journey, the fusion of yoga asana and Buddhist meditation—once viewed as heretical in both camps—has become common. It's hard to find a Buddhist retreat that doesn't offer the option of daily yoga or some other body-based practice; without it, the meditators might revolt. And yoga teachers routinely offer inspirational quotes from Buddhist masters in the midst of a sweaty *vinyasa* flow.

Over the years, countless students and fellow practitioners have told me that it was their practice of yoga asana that first opened the door for them to meditative awareness. When they first tried to practice seated meditation, their minds and hearts yearned for tranquility. But their nervous systems were jangled, their bodies were stressed, and they were disconnected from the embodied aliveness that provides fertile soil for meditative presence to grow. For them, the most direct and immediate doorway into mindful presence was through moving—and, more important, *feeling*—their physical bodies.

To understand why these body-based practices might be so important to contemporary meditators, let's do a little time travel together: imagine yourself as an aspiring yogi coming to meditation practice at the time of the Buddha, approximately five centuries B.C.E.

For your entire life, you have woken up and gone to sleep with the sun. You drink water from a nearby well or stream. If you want to go somewhere, you walk, bump along in a bullock cart, or—if you're very wealthy—ride a horse. You go barefoot most of the time or wear simple sandals. Most of your food is grown within a few miles of where you live—much of it, most likely, by you and your family. You're embedded in a web of clearly defined personal relationships, most of them with people you have known your entire life. You were born in your family home or a nearby field; you have burned your loved ones' bodies on funeral pyres and scattered their ashes in the same river where you wash your clothes. You don't know how to read, so you do not inhabit a world of abstract symbols. You inhabit a world of the physical senses—the smell of frangipani blossoms and cow dung, the taste of mustard and lentils, the sound of temple bells. You have never had a conversation with someone who is not physically present with you.

When you come to your meditation practice, your life is already grounded in the rhythms of your body and the earth in a way unknown to most modern, urbanized people except, perhaps, after weeks of wilderness backpacking. Your nervous system is moving at the pace of an oxcart. You do not reside primarily in your head—in fact, you are unfamiliar with the concept of the brain as an organ that generates thinking. (According to the best medical opinions of the time, the brain was an organ for filtering blood and generating mucus.) Your sense of "I" resides lower, at the center of your chest, where your heart is beating. In fact, your word for *heart* and *mind* is identical.

Now picture yourself as a person arriving at a meditation class or retreat today in a car that far outpaces the fastest horse of the Buddha's day—maybe even having flown there on a jet traveling thirty thousand feet above the earth's surface. Since waking up that morning, you have been bombarded with advertising messages and an estimated 34 gigabytes of information—just the latest day in a life that's probably been spent immersed in thinking, reading, and consuming media. You spend much of your workday communicating with people all over the world, many of whom you've never met, via phone, e-mail, and social networks. You eat your lunch while texting, monitoring several RSS feeds, and watching visceral video images of events on the other side of the globe. Your drinking water comes in plastic bottles labeled with pictures of distant snowcapped mountains.

And suddenly, you are asked to slam on your brakes, park your rear on a meditation cushion, and follow a system of sitting and walking that isn't much changed from the one followed by the Buddha's monks.

No wonder you feel a bit shell-shocked.

There's no way of knowing, of course, what it was really like for those early yogis. I don't want to romanticize life in ancient India, which contained, among other things, a staggering amount of oppression based upon social class, race, and gender.

But I venture that the typical person coming to a meditation practice today is jangled, disconnected, anxious, and trapped in his or her own head in a way that was virtually unheard of in the Buddha's time. The human organism may be fundamentally the same, but the level of stress, stimulation, and mental activity with which that organism has been pummeled is far greater.

For many contemporary practitioners, it's vital to have some way of reconnecting with their bodies and calming their nervous systems, just to come to the baseline sense of groundedness and ease that supports a deepening meditation practice. Mindfulness itself, of course, does not play favorites—in principle, we can be mindful of jangled nerves and careening thoughts just as well as we can be mindful of tranquility. But on a practical level, it can be easier to access our capacity for kind awareness—or even to remember that it exists—when there's some fundamental stability in the nervous system. For many of us, something other than just seated meditation is required.

But the reverse is also true: if your yoga practice consists only of the dynamic, flowing practice of physical postures that is the norm in most contemporary yoga classes, you are shortchanging yourself. The nonstop, ever-changing nature of an active physical practice—which is part of what makes it so engaging and entertaining—can distract you from turning your attention to the more subtle layers of your being. You will not be required to come face-to-face with the entrenched emotional and mental patterns that may be holding you hostage. And without the opportunity to simmer in them without distraction, you will not be able to liberate yourself from them.

To go deeper in your yoga, it's essential at some point that you *stop*, set up your body in a position that you can sustain for a while in relative comfort without falling asleep, and just *pay attention* for a while.

A DRIVE-BY TOUR OF YOGA HISTORY

"Mindful yoga" isn't just a random combination of techniques cooked up by marketing professionals to sell yoga wear. (*Get the new Mindfulness Camisole with built-in shelf bra!*) Buddhist mindfulness meditation and hatha yoga's postures and breathing techniques are different strands of the same braided rope of yogic history and philosophy. Like sisters growing up in the same intimate but occasionally quarrelsome family, these traditions have intermingled and influenced each other over centuries of interaction.

To explore the relationship between these two practices, let's pause for an abbreviated historical tour, a drive-by visit to a couple of key vista points in the vast and complex terrain of Indian philosophical and spiritual practice.

First Stop: Approximately 800 B.C.E.

In the humid jungles and river plains of what is now northeastern India flourishes a rigid, highly stratified theocracy dominated by a ruling elite of Brahman priests who serve as the intermediaries between human beings and the gods. The social fabric is stitched together by their ritual fires and animal sacrifices, which are believed to keep the cosmos from disintegrating, and which are celebrated in sacred hymns, known as the Vedas, that have been chanted aloud from generation to generation for hundreds of years.

However, on the fringes, growing numbers of spiritual seekers are dropping out. They're heading to snowbound Himalayan caves and jungles thick with elephants, tigers, and snakes to devote themselves to practices of mind and body that they hope will bring them into direct, personal contact with the luminous spirit that underlies all of life.

They shave their heads, dress in yellow robes and rags, live on handouts from villagers. And they wrestle with an eternal question that is still fresh for us today: How do human beings find lasting happiness in a world where nothing we love can last forever?

Rather than the external fires and sacrifices of the Brahman priests, these seekers cultivate the internal blaze of spiritual discipline, in which they immolate their past, their personal identities, and their attachments. They develop methods for entraining the mind into exquisitely blissful states of meditative absorption. At the core of their teachings is this: that at the heart of each human being is an eternal self that is inseparable from the eternal Self of the cosmos. And that it is possible for any human being to realize that oneness through a mind-training discipline that will eventually become known as yoga.

What You Need to Remember

Yogis and yoginis are radicals and explorers, experimenting in the laboratory of their own bodies and minds. The earliest yogis left behind family, work, and secular life to cultivate sophisticated methods for unifying the mind into deep, blissful states of meditative absorption.

Second Stop: Approximately 500 B.C.E.

In a remote province of northeastern India, the young son of a tribal chief gets wind of the teachings of these renegade yogis (despite the best efforts of his father to keep him away from them). Known to us now as Siddhartha Gotama (although this is probably a name ascribed to him later in history), this young man is a child of wealth and privilege, highly educated in philosophy, literature, and politics. He has a gorgeous wife and a young son and has been groomed to assume his place as a powerful local ruler in a part of India that is on the fringe of Brahmanical control. However, he has begun to question the meaning of all that he holds dear. How can he revel in his youthful body when old age, sickness, and death are inevitable? How can he enjoy his wealth when one day he'll have to leave it all behind? So one night he slips silently into his family's bedroom to take one last look at his sleeping wife and child. Then he shaves his head and joins the wandering yogis.

By this time these vagabond seekers have become a significant force in Indian society, which is in social and political upheaval. Packs of yellow-robed yogis travel from town to town and band together in forest communities. They migrate from one teacher to another, vigorously debating alternative approaches to dharma (truth) and ways of arriving at freedom from *dukkha,* the grinding sorrows and dissatisfactions of human life.

Siddhartha apprentices with several of the greatest yogis of his day, two of whom pronounce him a master of their arts and offer him leadership positions. However, although he rapidly achieves the states of meditative absorption that they teach, he notices that these states, though ecstatic, don't last. When he and the other yogis emerge from their meditative trances, they are plunged right back into a world of churning desires and unspeakable grief.

Leaving the ashrams, Siddhartha spends several years doing ascetic practices in a cave near Bodh Gaya, seeking to bully his body and mind into lasting freedom. He starves himself until his buttocks look like buffalo hooves and his backbone sticks out through the skin of his stomach. He holds his breath until his head throbs as if split with a sword. But eventually he rejects those methods, too, as not bringing durable happiness.

Finally, to the disgust of his fellow ascetics, he accepts a bowl of rice porridge from a village girl by the banks of a river and sits down on a grass cushion under a tree with heart-shaped leaves, vowing not to get up until he achieves full awakening. Seven days later, he succeeds in his quest and becomes known as the Buddha—a name that simply means "the Awakened One."

The Buddha's teachings have much in common with the yogic teachings that he has just departed from but are radically different in several important ways. Rather than positing union with an eternal Self as the doorway to liberation, the Buddha teaches that insight into the impermanent, ever-changing nature of all things—even the self—is the true freedom. Meditative concentration is to be used in the service of something called *sati,* a word that would come to be variously translated as "awareness," "mindfulness," or "remembering." For the Brahman priests, what is to be remembered are texts and scriptures. For the Buddha, what is to be remembered and tended to are the basic elements of the human experience: body, breath, heart, and mind.

The Buddha teaches for almost sixty years and leaves behind him a flourishing community of monks, nuns, and lay practitioners. Over the coming centuries, the Buddha's teachings will be carried on trade routes to China, Tibet, Southeast Asia, Japan—manifesting in each culture in a form appropriate for that time, that place, those people.

What You Need to Remember

The Buddha practiced and built upon the meditative arts cultivated by centuries of Indian yogis. He introduced the practice of mindfulness—turning the collected and unified attention to examine the arising and passing away of all phenomena. For the practice of mindfulness, you don't need to develop advanced states of deep meditative absorption. You just need to develop enough presence and stability of attention to see the true nature of what's happening inside you and all around you.

Third Stop: Approximately 200 C.E.

Since the time of the Buddha, his teachings have flourished in India in constant dialogue with other schools of yogic thought. Cross-pollination and -fertilization have been ongoing, as the yogic arts are living practice traditions, not rigid theoretical frameworks. One of these yogic paths is the system of *raja* or royal yoga (also known as *ashtanga* or eight-limbed yoga), which gets codified sometime between 200 B.C.E and 200 C.E. in a text called the Yoga Sutra, attributed to a sage named Patanjali, about whom very little is known.

In a series of terse aphorisms—clearly intended to be used as practice guides under the tutelage of a living master—Patanjali lays out an eight-pronged path for yogic awakening that includes many elements that are strikingly similar to the teachings of the Buddha, with which he was obviously familiar. Patanjali's yogic path begins with moral and ethical practices as its foundation. Upon this base the yogi assumes the posture of meditation—*asana*, a word that in this context literally means "seat"—and moves into pranayama: practices to cultivate and enhance the life force energy of prana through working with its physical manifestation, the breath. The yogi then progresses through the more and more subtle limbs of meditative practice, using the techniques of meditative absorption that were developed by many generations of yogis before the Buddha, which the Buddha himself utilized.

Patanjali does not mention the practice of mindfulness that is so central to the Buddha's teachings. However, his sutras directly point to the meditative ability to see clearly the nature of phenomena as they are—and thereby achieve freedom.

What You Need to Remember

Patanjali drew on and responded to the insights of generations of previous yogis, including the Buddha. He codified a path of yogic practice that includes the elements of ethics, body and breath disciplines, and successive stages of meditative absorption. This model of practice is still widely used in the yoga world today as a framework for understanding yogic disciplines.

Fourth Stop: 800–1100 C.E.—The Tantric Revolution

By "tantra" I'm not referring to the sexual techniques that spice up modern hot tub parties but to the multidimensional psycho-spiritual movement that sweeps through the Indian subcontinent in the second half of the first millennium and that has its roots in much more ancient shamanic practices. Emerging simultaneously in both Hindu and Buddhist schools of yoga, tantra serves as a potent counterpose to the ascetic view that has begun to dominate both of those traditions.

Previously the teachings of all the great yogis—including the Buddha and Patanjali—were unified around a common goal: to see reality clearly and thereby arrive at inner freedom. But in their zeal to break free of painful clinging to an impermanent world, many yogic lineages, both Buddhist and Hindu, had calcified around a rejection not just of the body—impermanent and filled with insatiable desires—but of everything associated with it: sexuality, women, family life, the earth, incarnation itself.

But tantra is a grassroots movement whose earliest adepts are not monks but householders, often from the lowest castes of Indian society—fishermen, wine sellers, washerwomen, and cow herders, people whose days are dipped in the grittiest details of the physical world. To the tantrika, this ever-changing world of ocean, wine, soap suds, and manure is a manifestation of the eternal, formless absolute and, hence, is not an obstacle to awakening but a vehicle for it. And so, by extension, is human flesh. In their celebration of all aspects of birth and death—whether ecstatic or horrific—tantrikas shatter societal convention and ritualize taboos: drinking alcohol, eating meat, having sex unsanctioned by marriage, wandering naked in garbage heaps and charnel grounds.

From this fertile brew of ideas and practices emerges hatha yoga—the systematic art of using the body as a tool for liberation. Hatha yoga shares tantra's elaborate mapping of the subtle body—an intricate network of energies coursing through channels called *nadis* and concentrated in swirling vortexes called chakras. The intense physical techniques of hatha yoga are a kind of ritual alchemy through which these energies can be harnessed for liberation. Hatha yoga adepts codify their discoveries in a series of texts that include the classic Gheranda Samhita and Hatha Yoga Pradipika.

With their matted hair, ash-covered bodies, and association with tantric techniques, hatha yogis quickly get a bad rap in contemporary Indian society, which associates them with black magic. But hatha yogis insist that, in fact, they are practicing a version of Patanjali's raja yoga—which becomes their "cover story" distinguishing them from their tantric peers. Their postures, they proclaim, are just elaborations on Patanjali's asana, or meditative seat. In the Buddhist tradition, the tantric practices of yoga postures and breath work become incorporated into the form of Buddhism that is developing in Tibet—known as *vajrayana*.

Whether you are standing on your head, pouring salt water into your sinuses, or swallowing a piece of cloth and then hauling it out of your stomach again—you have to perform these physical practices in the service of ultimate spiritual awakening, hatha yogis say, or your actions are meaningless. At the same time, hatha yoga's body-based techniques keep the practitioner grounded in the world of physical form—the only place where it is possible to honor the preciousness of human incarnation, with its infinite sorrows and infinite joys.

What You Need to Remember

Hatha yoga's elaborate asanas and breathing techniques are a relative newcomer to the yoga tool kit. They're meant to be used as a support for meditation and as an expression of it—a way to ground in and honor the incarnate world of form as well as the formless Absolute.

Fifth Stop: Twentieth Century c.e.

In the early 1900s in India there is a revival of interest in the art of hatha yoga, which mainstream Indian culture has long viewed with suspicion as the province of matted-hair dropouts from respectable society. Indian nationalists want to cultivate an indigenous health and fitness system to counter the YMCA model imported by the British. Yogic pioneers begin digging out ancient hatha yoga texts, combining their methods with Western gymnastics and fitness systems, and presenting them in a sanitized modern context—as methods for cultivating wellness and vitality of body, mind, and spirit. One of these yogic pioneers, T. Krishnamacharya, allegedly travels to Tibet to study yoga with Tibetan Buddhist masters and incorporates their living tradition into the fusion of yogic philosophy and Western gymnastics that he teaches to the princes at the Mysore Palace.

Western seekers begin traveling to India and studying these repackaged yogic systems with teachers such as B. K. S. Iyengar, Swami Satchidananda, and many others. They bring them back to the United States, where they merge with a flourishing health, fitness, and personal-growth movement. At the same time, Buddhist meditative traditions from widely different cultures—Tibetan, Thai, Japanese, Vietnamese—begin taking root in the West as well. Japanese Zen masters sent to the United States to minister to the needs of Japanese congregations find themselves heading up communes launched by their young hippie followers. Thai forest monks teach Peace Corps workers and draft dodgers.

In the late twentieth century, hatha yoga's physical postures and breathing practices are repackaged as a popular fitness and stress-reduction practice that attracts tens of millions of practitioners. While some of these practitioners are content to keep their yoga practice as a stress-busting workout, many others become curious about its deeper potential.

These modern yogis and yoginis have access to a wide range of tools and techniques that have developed in different epochs, different cultures, different countries—but share the ancient yogic goal of liberation from suffering by meditative awakening to the truth of how things are. Practitioners move fluidly from yoga workouts with a world-beat sound track to ten-day silent vipassana retreats, from a stress-reduction meditation course prescribed by their doctor to a Zen intensive led by a shaven-head priest who is also a soccer mom.

What You Need to Remember

Yoga today is part of a living tradition, constantly innovating—while in dialogue with other living traditions—to meet the needs of each new generation of practitioners.

Final Stop: You

Yogis have always been supremely practical, picking up whatever tool is needed to bring about liberation.

As you step on your mat or sit on your meditation cushion, as you listen to alignment cues from an asana instructor or to a dharma talk from a Buddhist monk, you're not doing two separate practices. You're engaged in different aspects of the same practice, picking up different tools from the ancient and evolving yogic tool kit.

Like the ancient yogis, you're seeking out the best teachings available from a wide range of traditions. Like them, you're engaged in a delicate balance of respecting tradition and innovating and synthesizing to create a system that works for your culture, your body, your times.

Externally, your quest may look different: while they went into forests and caves, you are going to ashrams, yoga studios, and retreat centers. But on the internal level, you're doing exactly what they ultimately had to do: you're heading into the wilderness of your own body and mind, the uncharted territory of your own psyche. And you're engaged in the eternal yogic questions: How do I live with this human body? How do I live with this human mind? These are questions that can be answered only in *your* body, in *your* life.

Now is the first word of Patanjali's Yoga Sutra: *Atha yoga anushasanam: Now, the practice of yoga.* Five hundred years before that, the Buddha taught, "Do not pursue the past. Do not lose yourself in the future. The past no longer is. The future has not yet come."

This is what every yogi and mystic discovers: the present moment is a doorway into the infinite. And not just some *special* present moment, *this* one. Any moment will do. The *now* of Patanjali has become our *then,* just as the Buddha's future unfurled into Patanjali's present. The Yoga Sutra was chanted aloud for hundreds of years before it was written down on palm-leaf paper that has long since crumbled away. What was the *now* of Patanjali, whoever he was? A patter of monsoon rain on jungle palms? The cool, sweet taste of a mango? The texts attributed to Patanjali and the Buddha are fossils. To see the living flower of the teachings burst into bloom, you have to do the practice yourself.

■◀ To experience a short guided mindfulness meditation, go to annecushman.com/practices.

CHAPTER 3

The Art of Practice

WHILE I WAS MEDITATING early one morning a few years ago, my then eight-year-old son Skye came into my room. I got off my cushion and got back into bed to snuggle and chat—about the day ahead, his dreams, my dreams. The bell on my phone chimed three times.

"What's that?" he asked.

"It's my meditation timer," I told him.

He looked bewildered. "If meditation is just about being present for every moment," he asked, "then why do you need a *timer?*"

Well, okay, in theory you don't. But in practice it's good to carve out a special time and place for your practice. It's a window into your life—a place where you can touch what it is to be human and practice the art of being alive. It's a glass-bottomed boat through which you can cruise on your own inner tropical ocean, peering down at strange and beautiful fish.

The program in this book will work best if you are willing to set aside regular time—ideally, every day—to take these miniretreats to cultivate the practices and principles it contains. While it's great to go to a guided class, there's no substitute for a personal home practice in which you can explore your body and heart at your own pace, under your own direction.

For many people a home practice is challenging. Many of us have cultivated our yoga asana practice almost entirely in the context of a guided class. We're used to an external voice continually telling us what to do with our bodies and where to focus our attention. The teacher's voice is like a sheepdog nipping at the heels of the wandering flock of our thoughts. Without it they run off into the hills, lost and bleating.

But that's precisely why it's so useful to practice on your own. Even if your mind appears to wander more and your practice initially feels less focused, each time you kindly bring your attention back to the *now* of your practice—*on your own,* without an external reminder— you train up your capacity for compassionate presence. In your daily life, you don't have a teacher's soothing voice coaching you moment to moment to stay in your body; you have to remember on your own. So a home practice offers you the opportunity to practice again and again—and *again* and *again*—that returning to the ever-shifting center of your body-heart-mind.

You could spend hours planning a time in the future when you will finally be able to connect with the present moment. You could go online and research various retreat centers. You could buy a travel yoga mat, a folding wooden meditation bench, a new yoga outfit. Request the vacation time from your boss, arrange the child care, buy the tickets, pack the suitcase.

Or you could just turn to your home practice—and be present right now. A daily home practice can be like a miniretreat in the middle of your life—a retreat of an hour or a half hour, a retreat of five minutes or five breaths. I once heard the Zen teacher Thich Nhat Hanh say that these oases of practice should not be called retreats— they should be called *treats.* They're a time for a pilgrimage into the wilderness of your own body and heart to see what reveals itself and to take whatever shows up as your teacher—an aching back, a worn-out argument, a moment of joy as darting and bright as a hummingbird.

Here are some reflections around common questions that come up about structuring a daily practice of mindful yoga and meditation.

WHEN SHOULD I PRACTICE?

Back before I had a child, in my twenties and early thirties, I used to keep a fire wall around my practice to keep it separate from the routine conflagrations of my life. I always practiced first thing in the morning, before I did anything else. For two hours I would leave my phone unplugged. I wouldn't speak to my housemates or even my cat.

But after I had a baby, all of that changed. I learned to practice in stolen moments while he was preoccupied with his mobile. My asanas unfolded in five-minute intervals, accompanied by the tinkling sound of his musical toys: *How much is that doggie in the window?* . . .

With time, my practice has gotten more porous and fluid. I carve out the time each day wherever I can find it—sometimes early morning, sometimes just before lunch, sometimes late in the evening before I go to sleep.

It does help to pick a time of the day when you can be regular and consistent. Be realistic—don't set yourself up for failure by committing yourself to more than you can do. But do what it takes to make it happen. Set the alarm fifteen minutes early. Or stay up half an hour after everyone else is in bed. Make it a date with yourself, as if you were making a plan with your best friend. Mark it on your calendar or program an alarm into your phone.

View your practice as a gift to yourself, not a burden. It's your time to listen to that soft inner voice that gets drowned out by the rest of daily life. It is your time to be a diver, swimming down into your depths to find the shimmering pearls.

But the journey is not about bringing the pearls to the surface to wear them or sell them. It's about the swimming itself, the coral reefs and sea monsters you see along the way.

So be firm about setting aside your practice time, but also be flexible. Remember that life is not an interruption of practice. On a spiritual pilgrimage to India, I was shocked to discover how much of my time was spent washing out dirty socks and underwear in a sink and hanging them to dry on a portable travel line stretched between a bed slat and a doorknob, or walking down grubby alleys looking for Imodium and toothpaste. These so-called interruptions, I finally realized, were in fact what the pilgrimage was all about.

WHERE SHOULD I PRACTICE?

According to the Hatha Yoga Pradipika, to do your yoga practice properly, you need a small hermitage whose walls are patted down regularly with cow dung.

If, like most of us, you can't swing a cave or a hermitage—or even a whole separate room—just set aside a corner of the living room or bedroom. Do your best to make it somewhere peaceful and serene, where the space itself supports the mental state that you want to be cultivating. Consider a flower or a stick of incense to delight the senses. Make it as inviting as a bed with fresh silk sheets or a candlelit table beautifully set for one.

Put something in your practice space that inspires you: a statue or a sculpture or a painting. Have the things that you need stored tidily nearby: a rolled-up mat, a few folded blankets, a couple of yoga belts, a meditation cushion. But don't be fanatical about it. Your wild and woolly life will bleed in around the edges, and that's okay. You're not becoming perfect. You're becoming more yourself.

I have to confess: my practice space is also my bedroom, so before I practice I generally have to toss a pile of dirty laundry into a basket before I can roll out my mat. But that is just life. We all have to practice in the middle of our dramas, and sometimes that gets messy. We just have to clear the space for it.

WHAT SHOULD I PRACTICE?

For some people—on some days—what's called for is a sweaty power vinyasa followed by a long Savasana. For other people—on other days—what's needed is just to drape their bodies over some bolsters for a few restorative poses and then to meditate on a bench in the garden.

Because the essence of a mindful yoga practice is deep listening, I hesitate to get too prescriptive. However, as a general guideline, while working through the program in this book, think of your formal daily practice as having three main components:

1. Exploring and cultivating the physical body through meditation-in-movement (asana)
2. Exploring and cultivating the breath and energy body (pranayama)
3. Exploring and cultivating the mind and heart in the seated meditation posture or some other posture that can be held for long periods in stillness

For each week of this twelve-week course, I'll give methods for these three dimensions of formal practice—as well as suggestions for taking your explorations off the mat and cushion and into your life. However, some weeks will emphasize one aspect of the practice more than another, as we highlight different facets of the jewel of compassionate mindfulness.

If you're a yoga practitioner, you're probably familiar with the classical sequencing of these elements in the order they are listed in Patanjali's Yoga Sutra: first asana, then pranayama, then the various stages of meditation. It's a logical sequence that reflects a natural interiorization of our attention from the denser, more easily felt and guided layers of our being to the more subtle energetic, emotional, and mental dimensions. For most of us, it's easiest to focus our attention first on the physical form. Once our attention is stabilized, we can start investigating less tangible aspects of our experience without getting lost or swept away.

But, in fact, this progression is less a linear sequence than an ever-deepening spiral. And the more deeply you go into your practice, the more you'll find that the distinctions between these practices reveal themselves as somewhat arbitrary. Each of these practices contains elements of all of the others, and the boundaries between them are fluid. How can you move the body without breathing? How can you examine the breath without studying the mind that flows along with it? A seated meditation position is simply another yoga posture— remember that the original meaning of the word *asana* is literally "seat." The intimate connection with the breath that you develop in pranayama is a form of meditation. And as soon as you tend the garden of your asana practice, you encounter the thorns and blossoms of your heart-mind.

So, for every week I'll give you suggestions, but don't be rigid. Feel free to begin with whatever is calling you most: a series of vigorous Sun Salutations; a long, restorative back bend draped over a pile of bolsters; some alternate-nostril breathing. Some days you may want to sit in meditation before you start to move. Create enough structure to support your practice, but then be flexible. Let your unfolding practice guide you from inside.

PART TWO   Twelve Weeks

Inhabiting Your Body

IN THE EARLY 1990s I journeyed to interview the yoga master B. K. S. Iyengar at his yoga institute in Pune, India—a trip that for a modern hatha yogi is something like a devout Muslim's pilgrimage to Mecca. I rattled by auto rickshaw through the choking fumes of downtown Pune to the institute—housed in a modest building in a quiet residential neighborhood, with a statue near the entrance of Iyengar balanced on one leg in Natarajasana, the Dancer's Pose.

Inside, the bright, airy practice room was jammed with fifty or sixty people in an array of supported postures: draped over bolsters, suspended from wall ropes, strapped to wooden horses, buried under sandbags and immense iron disks. From my perch in a corner stairwell, I watched as the seventy-nine-year-old Iyengar, his immense torso swelling over his shorts, darted through the room like a sheepdog corralling a flock: growling, barking, offering lightning-quick adjustments with a tug here, a slap there.

Catching sight of me, he strode over. "You journalists! You say that asana practice is only physical! But where is the spiritual person who does not have a body?" He glowered at me. "You understand nothing!"

A few days later we sipped chai together in his library—his apparent rage forgotten—and he told me more about just how vital his decades-long exploration of the art of asana was to his spiritual survival. When he turned sixty, he said, his guru—the renowned Sri

Krishnamacharya—told him it was time to stop doing asanas and focus on meditation practice instead. Obediently, Iyengar stopped his asana practice for three months. "What was the effect? I lost everything. Three months, and it's taken me years to come back to life."

Iyengar leaned toward me, his eyes drilling into mine. "Now, if God himself were to come to me and tell me, 'Leave the asana practice behind!' I would say to God, 'NO! I will not leave it.'"

Many of us hatha yogis can relate to Iyengar's passion for his asana practice. Because on the path of hatha yoga, our bodies are our gateway to the infinite. They may be the place where we first sensed what it was to be vibrantly present and alive or where we slowly groped our way back to a connection with our hearts.

And in the teachings of the Buddha, mindfulness of the body—directly sensing our bodies with loving awareness just as they are in the present moment—is fundamental to the path of awakening. It's the first of what he called the Four Foundations of Mindfulness, the four arenas of our human experience in which we can cultivate the art of being fully present and see into the true nature of ourselves and the world.

But even the phrasing "mindfulness of the body" is deceptive—implying that you are somehow separate from your body, tending it from a distance, like a babysitter watching a toddler digging in a sandbox. What you'll be exploring this week is a way of coming alive in your body from the inside, so you're right there digging in the sand yourself.

This week we will lay the foundation for our practice of mindful yoga and embodied meditation by cultivating the powerful, and deceptively simple, art of fully inhabiting the ever-changing stream of sensation that we call a body. We'll discover a relationship with our physical form that serves awakening and freedom. We'll learn to be in touch with our bodies without being identified with them.

And when we practice this way, all the rest of the Buddha's teachings can come alive for us from the inside out—not as a concept or another set of admonitions about how to be good but as embodied understanding.

■◖ For a guided yoga and meditation session based on the principles in this chapter, go to annecushman.com/practices.

The Body-Mind Matrix

In the yoga tradition, the physical body is known as the *annamaya-kosha*—literally, the "meat body." This physical *kosha* (body) is viewed as just one dimension of our multilayered being. Yogis described our physical body as surrounded and permeated by our *pranamayakosha* (breath and energy body), *manomayakosha* (mental and emotional body), *vijnanamayakosha* (wisdom body), and *anandamayakosha* (bliss body). These koshas are not separate layers, like the layers of an onion; they are a fluid continuum of matter and energy. From the yogic perspective, what we think of as *mind* and what we think of as *body* are different vibrations of the same spectrum.

Mind and body are also inseparable from the perspective of modern science. Our thoughts and emotions both emerge from the complex interaction of mutually interdependent physical systems—the firing of neurons, the release of hormones—and, in turn, shape the way those systems unfold.

Therefore, when you work with your physical body, you are directly influencing your heart and mind. You don't have to buy into the yogic cosmology of koshas, or become an expert on neuroscience, to experience this directly. All you have to do is get a massage when you're stressed out and watch how your anxiety melts away along with the knots in your neck muscles.

And the physical body has the advantage of being the densest, most easily contacted manifestation of our multilayered being. As the great bodyworker Ida Rolf once said, "I know the body isn't all that there is—but it's all that I can get my hands on." By getting intimately connected with our bodies, we can open the door to a deeper, more sensitive, and more skillful connection with all the other levels of our being.

WHY IS MINDFULNESS OF THE BODY IMPORTANT?

Here are just a few of the reasons that grounding your attention in your body is vital to the practice of awakening.

1. *Your body is always right here, right now.* This transient, mysterious body anchors you in the beauty or sorrow of each unfolding moment: the smell of piñon logs blazing in a woodstove, your grandmother's frail hand in yours as you say good-bye. And it's only when you're present for these moments that it's possible to be intimate with your life.

If you're already a yoga practitioner, this may strike you as old news at first. If you practice yoga regularly, you've got a head start in terms of physical awareness that will serve you well in your meditation practice. You're familiar with paying attention to the fine details of your body and breath: from the placement of your little toe to the length of your inhalation.

But even yoga can be done on autopilot. (At this point in my practice, I'm perfectly capable of going through a whole series of Sun Salutations while rehearsing my day's to-do list.) And when we're engaged in an active asana practice, we often feel in the service of *doing.* We sense the base of our skull—in order to lift it. We sense the space between the shoulder blades—in order to broaden it. Sometimes it's easier to feel the body when we're actively moving it, which is why yoga asana can be a useful tool. But if that's all we're capable of, it has ceased to be a tool and become a crutch.

It's one thing to feel our bodies when we are pounding them with intense sensation through dramatic physical postures. But can we feel them when the movements and sensations are more subtle? How about when they're not moving at all? Can we be as fascinated with the subtle movement of breath in the belly for forty minutes as we can be with forty minutes of rigorous vinyasa?

Often we come to yoga because we want our body to be different. We want to be fifteen pounds thinner. We want to be flexible and gorgeous like the person on the next mat.

But a mindful practice is not primarily about getting somewhere else. It's about opening to where you actually are—to what's true for your real body, your real life. It's about entering into the realm of your senses: hearing the rain on the roof and the *swish* of car tires in the puddles, smelling the soured milk and lemon peel in the garbage disposal.

2. *Your physical body is inextricably connected with your breath, your heart, and your mind.* So when you ground your practice in your body, you enhance your ability to investigate other aspects of your experience through your meditative attention—your energy, your emotions, your thoughts, your relationships—not as abstract ideas but as felt experiences.

   As we'll explore in depth in weeks 3 and 4, the breath is commonly used as a focal point for meditation. Feeling your breath from the inside as a sensuous, full-body experience is very different from—and for many people, more compelling than—mentally focusing on it as if watching it from the outside. As this program progresses, you'll build on the body sensitivity you cultivate this week to heighten your awareness of more and more subtle dimensions of your experience, including the attitude you hold toward yourself and others.

3. *Your body sensations can be a focal point around which to gather and unify a scattered mind.* In the Satipatthana Sutta, the classic teaching on the Four Foundations of Mindfulness, the Buddha instructed his monks and nuns to know their bodies "up from the soles of their feet and down from the top of the hair," connecting with precise attention to everything from skin, teeth, and kidneys to pus, bile, and feces. He urged them to contemplate their bodies from the inside and from the outside, knowing each part with the specificity of a person sorting through a sack of many sorts of grains: "hill rice, red rice, beans, peas, millet."

   As you learn to focus your attention this way in some specific aspect of your direct experience of your body, you are cultivating the art of what's known in Pali as *samatha*. *Samatha* is frequently translated as "concentration," but in English that word brings the unfortunate connotation of mental strain. What we are talking about is concentration in the sense that an extract of vanilla is concentrated flavor—undiluted. Rather than your attention's being dispersed, it is gathered together and unified, and like the flavor of vanilla extract, it becomes more powerful. When focused in the body, this kind of concentration is not a mental effort but an intensification of a felt sense of presence. In meditation, concentration works hand in hand with mindfulness. In week 5, we'll investigate further into the relationship between these two dimensions of meditative practice.

4. *Your body reveals that everything arises and passes away.* As you settle your attention in your body, an important truth becomes obvious: it's always changing. Each time you come to your mat or cushion, you're inhabiting a slightly different body: tighter or looser, lighter or heavier, sleepier or more energetic. And as your attention becomes more refined, what you thought was solid—a foot, a hip, a hand—reveals itself as an evanescent flow of sensations that you can influence but not control.

In modern Westernized culture, we have a strange relationship with our bodies: simultaneously desperately attached to them and profoundly out of touch with them. We're afraid to inhabit them fully, but we want to control them, we want them to look good, and we definitely want them to last forever.

If we're not careful, this attitude can insidiously creep into our yoga practice as well. Our practice can become focused on looking and feeling good to the exclusion of all else. It's true that the hatha yoga tradition is, among other things, a potent tool kit for physical health and well-being. Pick up any popular yoga magazine and you'll find a plethora of ways to use yoga to feel or look better: Yoga for insomnia. Yoga for flatter abs. Yoga for back pain, core strength, stress reduction, more and better orgasms.

There's nothing unspiritual about such health and fitness pursuits. A strong, healthy body is a powerful support for a spiritual practice; a weak, addicted, or pain-ridden one can be a powerful distraction.

The problem arises when we become attached to physical well-being as an end in itself and to our yoga practice as the ultimate fix-it kit. Because sooner or later, each of us is going to encounter a physical condition or life situation that just can't be fixed. We're going to meet the illness that can't be cured, the grief that can't be mended, the death of someone we love. How do we practice with our bodies in a way that prepares us to lose them in the end—along with everything else we hold dear? This is the territory of a mindful yoga practice—a practice that honors our body as sacred while also bringing home the truth that it won't be here forever.

How I Learned to Feel My Body

As the daughter of a Catholic army general, I grew up on military posts with cannons decorating the street corners, armed guards at the gates, and soldiers saluting our family car. "Feel your body" is not an instruction that is often given to soldiers—or, for that matter, to the nuns who taught my sixth-grade class at Immaculate Conception elementary school.

When I began doing yoga, at first it took a lot of large, strong, vigorous movements for me to feel anything at all—vigorous vinyasa and dramatic poses that could smash through the concrete that had paved me over so I could feel the small, delicate sprouts of sensation that wanted to come up through the cracks. I needed to have my joints hammered, my muscles yanked—to sweat and puff my way to that blissful buzz that saturated every cell with aliveness.

Gradually, my armor melted. I began to savor the subtle sensations of a joint turning in a socket, a patch of skin sliding a millimeter in one direction or another, the breath traveling up the inner wall of the nostrils and out down the outer wall. I began to come alive to my senses. With time, I learned to love to practice slowly so I could feel sensations bloom in my body in exquisite slow motion.

And when I remember to live my life like that, everything starts to sing—like the soup of white bean and kale I made for my dinner last night with thyme, rosemary, and tomatoes straight from my garden. The soup sang to me of the farmers who planted the onion and the garlic and of the people who drove the trucks that carried them to the store. It sang of the day last spring when we planted the tomatoes—Skye and I on our knees in the garden bed, dark earth under our fingernails, the sun on our backs. It sang of worms burrowing deep into the earth—and of the earth itself, formed of particles forged in ancient, exploded stars.

REDISCOVERING RELIEF ⟡ Nathalie Bittar

Born in Beirut, Lebanon, Nathalie Bittar runs Blue Nile Yoga Center in Khartoum, Sudan.

I don't publicize the yoga studio; it's very much word of mouth. But the classes are packed. The folks here don't have other places where they're given freedom to move creatively, to sit in silence in darkness where no one knows them and where they are able to hear what is going on in their minds and bodies. It's a relief for them. It reminds them of something that they have forgotten.

One of the students says that for her, the yoga and meditation are a way of cleansing before prayer, a method of arriving at a place of stillness from which she can access Allah more directly.

Most of the women have practiced very few sports. The physical asanas allow the women to move into their bodies. With not much exposure to physical exercises, simple poses like Happy Baby Pose elicit unexpected bursts of laughter. Their bodies experience these new forms, creating a shock, and at the same time a magical experience. They love very simple poses, like Child's Pose. A gentle head massage in Savasana and they melt and relax.

Yoga gives them permission to get to know their bodies, to start to actually feel their bodies. From there a lot of things open up. In meditation they uncover a safe place where there is no social pressure and from where they have permission to listen to what's coming up without judgment or reaction. They tap into a still space where they find refuge regardless of the social or political instabilities surrounding them. This gives them a new sense of power.

WEEK 1 PRACTICES

When developing mindfulness in an asana practice, it's easy to default to a familiar, goal-oriented focus because of all the complex and sometimes demanding actions that are required. So in our practices this week, we will primarily train our ability to sense and inhabit our body either in stillness or in very simple movements designed to awaken sensation. In week 2 we will build on this awareness by extending it into more traditional asanas.

Spend anywhere from 15 to 60 minutes each day exploring one or more of this week's body-sensing practices.

Begin every asana practice session with practice 1.1: Arriving in Your Body. From there, practices 1.2, 1.3A, 1.3B, 1.3C, 1.4, and 1.5 are all ways to deepen your connection with your body before moving into more active asanas.

Your most important practice this week, though, is practice 1.5: Exploring the Whole Body. At least 3 or 4 times this week, take 25 to 30 minutes to do this entire body-sensing practice, followed by at least 5 to 15 minutes of seated meditation.

These practices blossom with regular repetition over time. And each time you revisit one of them, you're stepping into a different river. It's like getting to know a new friend: you don't find out everything about the person on your first lunch date. It takes time to cultivate a meaningful relationship.

Do not be fooled by the simplicity of this week's practices; they are immensely powerful. The sensitivity to your inner world that you cultivate will be the foundation of all further practice and will only deepen over weeks and months and years of repetition. Like secret messages written in invisible ink, dimensions of your being that you were unaware of will shimmer into view.

And as you become more attuned to the bare sensations of your physical experience, you'll have access to direct sensing of your mental, emotional, and energetic life as well—all of which will directly serve you as you continue your investigation into what creates suffering for you and what leads you to peace, joy, and true liberation.

Perhaps most important, you will become more and more sensitive to the spacious awareness in which all of your body sensations arise and pass away. You'll learn to feel your body vividly while simultaneously knowing that your true nature is vaster and more luminous than its fragile web of bone, blood, sinew, and skin.

PRACTICE 1.1
Arriving in Your Body (3–5 minutes)

This is a great way to begin any practice session.

Sit, stand, or lie down in a comfortable position that you can sustain for several minutes without squirming or shifting. Let your eyes close. Then extend an invitation to yourself to come home to your body.

First of all, notice: Where in your body are you living right now? If your body were a house, would you be up in the attic of your head, perhaps pressed up against the window of your eyes straining to look out? Are you huddled around a pain or injury in some cramped corner? Melt your attention down out of your head and throughout your body, as if draining your brain. Along the way, sense and soften around any obvious areas that might be holding pain or tension: the muscles around the eyes, the hinge of your jaw, the root of your tongue, your belly, your pelvic floor. Relax any gripping that pulls your body away from the support of the earth. Notice whether your breath changes as you take up residence lower and lower in your body.

If it helps you descend, place one hand on your heart and the other on your belly and let the contact of your hands magnetize your attention. Can you feel your way all the way into your pelvic floor? How about the soles of your feet?

How is your body feeling today? Sluggish? Buzzing with energy? Bloated? Tingling with pleasure? Are there areas that seem lit up in your attention because they feel so good or because they hurt? What rooms in your body do you have easy access to? What rooms are locked?

Don't worry if whole sectors seem cordoned off from your explorations. Right now you're just doing a preliminary survey of your inner territory. You'll have plenty of time to take up residence as your practice unfolds.

PRACTICE 1.2
Waking Up Sensation with Movement (5–15 minutes)

In most of this week's practices, you'll be sensing the body in stillness so as not to get distracted by habitual patterns of doing and achieving. However, for many people it can be hard at first to feel the body without a little bit of action. This practice is a good way to flow into either a more active asana practice or one of the other sensing practices below. I particularly like to do this practice lying down, but you can also do it sitting or standing.

You can begin anywhere in your body that you have some mobility—your left big toe, your right index finger, the tip of your tailbone—wherever is calling you. However, I'll use your shoulder as an example.

Begin with the Arriving in Your Body practice (page 38). When you've completed it, let your attention flow into your right shoulder. Inhabit your shoulder joint with your attention, fully taking up residence. Then begin to move your shoulder in a free-form, nontechnical way. Roll your shoulder forward and back, up and down, in big and little circles and spirals. Sense the intricate dance of shoulder blades, upper arm bone, collarbone. Don't worry if your mind isn't clear on the names or shapes of the anatomical structures. Create your own inner map based purely on sensation.

Now let the shoulder relax, and invite your awareness to travel down into your elbow. Flex and extend the arm, waking up sensation in that joint. The range of motion of the elbow joint is less than that of the shoulder—does that mean the sensations are less vibrant as well?

Traverse your arm down into your wrist. Flex, extend, roll—sense from the inside what your wrist can do. Then continue to travel out through the hand, furling and unfurling the fingers like flower petals. Can you enliven every joint of every finger?

Now let the whole arm wriggle and writhe like a snake. Sense the arm extending from roots deep in your heart, or even your belly, all the way out to the very tips of your finger. Let the free-form movements heighten your ability to feel your arm. When you have finished, let the arm relax by your side. Sense the difference between that arm and the other.

From your right arm, move on to the left arm. Then continue to your legs: Is it easier for you to start your movement explorations with the hip? Or are your toes more accessible at first? Then investigate your spine, beginning at the tip of your tailbone or at your atlas vertebra, deep in your skull. What kinds of undulations and oscillations help you live inside your spine?

Continue this exploration until you have "woken up" your entire body with gentle, nondemanding movement.

From here you are ready to flow into the rest of your asana practice or to refine and heighten your awareness with some of the other body-sensing practices below.

PRACTICE 1.3A
Feel Your Hand (3–5 minutes)

When you sustain your continuous attention in any part of your body, it comes alive in your awareness as living sensation, far more nuanced than your mental images of it. Because they're so sensitive and dense with nerve endings— and, for most people, not particularly emotionally loaded—your hands are a good place to explore this, but you can try this exercise with any body part.

In this and all of the other awareness practices in this chapter, it's important not to strain to track down sensations. Let the sensations come to you rather than chasing after them. Whatever you are feeling is exactly right. Remember: You're not in a hurry.

Sit in any comfortable position—on a chair, on the floor, on a cushion, in a parked car, or wherever you happen to be. Set a timer to ring in 3 to 5 minutes. Hold out your left hand, palm up or down, and hover it a few inches above your leg.

Look at your hand, studying it from the outside—the shape of the fingers, the color and texture of the skin. Now close your eyes and invite your attention to move into your internal experience of your hand. Not your mental picture of your hand—the actual feeling, from the inside out. How is this different from viewing it from the outside? This direct, sensate knowing of your physical experience is sometimes referred to as the "felt sense" of your body, and it is central to an embodied practice of meditation.

How do you know you have a hand? Is there a feeling of heaviness, lightness? Tingling? Pulsing? Can you feel the back of the hand? The palm of your hand? The air on your skin? The space between the fingers? Beneath the fingernails? Between the bones? Is the skin on your hand damp or dry? Hot or cool?

Notice whether you are reflexively turning your eyes behind your eyelids to look at your hand. Instead, soften the eyes and relax into feeling. Notice your sense of the hand developing like a Polaroid photo, getting more and more multilayered and nuanced. Remember, this is a meditation practice—you're cultivating the art of focusing and stabilizing your mind. And as with any meditation training, your mind will inevitably wander. When this happens, just coax it back home to the felt sense of your hand.

By the time the timer rings, your hand may be bursting with sensation, like fireworks of feeling going off in the sky of your awareness.

Now ask yourself: Were these sensations there all along, though you have only just started noticing them? Or did you create the sensations with the power of your focused attention?

Try this: Do this practice with your foot. Try it once with the foot flat on the ground, either standing or sitting. Then try it lying down with the leg extended, so the sole of the foot is open to the air. Are these different experiences? How does your attention change in your foot when it's in a weight-bearing position?

PRACTICE 1.3B
Feel Both Hands (3–5 Minutes)

Now you'll explore the fluid quality of your focused attention—the way it can flow from one object to another while remaining soft and receptive. You can move into this practice directly from practice 1.3A or do it as a stand-alone practice.

Just as you did in the previous exercise, sit comfortably with your eyes closed, hover your right hand (palm up or down), and fully inhabit it with your attention.

Now lift your left hand and hover it as well, with the palm facing the same way as the right one. Gradually flow your attention from the right hand into the left. Does it leap there right away? Or does it trickle there like honey? Let the right hand fade into the background, and take all the time you need to inhabit your left.

Now pour the attention slowly back and forth from one hand to the other. Does one hand fade out gradually as the other fades in? Or do they blink in and out of focus right from the start? Notice whether there's a dualistic sense of viewing the hands from the outside, as mental images— as if *you* and *hand* are two separate entities. Instead, inhabit the hands from the inside out, as if the hands were coming alive to themselves.

Finally, see if you can sense both hands simultaneously. When you do that, does your attention diffuse or do the details of each hand remain crisp? Are you truly holding them both at the same time, or are you flickering rapidly back and forth?

When you sense both hands at the same time, what happens to your thoughts?

Try this: Do this practice with your feet.

PRACTICE 1.3C
Focus the Lens of Awareness (3–5 minutes)

After you've gotten fluent in the language of sensation in practices 1.3A and 1.3B, experiment with the focus of your lens. Playing with the lens of awareness is a crucial skill for meditation practice. Notice how natural it is. Your lens is always shifting in response to your inner and outer circumstances. In mindfulness practice, you learn to make that process conscious so you have more choice about where you place your attention.

Hover one hand as in practice 1.3A. First dial the lens in tight: Just sense your forefinger. Now just the tip of your forefinger. Now just the sensation under the fingernail. How laser-like can you make your attention? Take your time. Move from one tiny area to another: the webbing between your thumb and first finger; the mound at the root of the ring finger. Notice whether you are tensing the muscles around your eyes in an attempt to concentrate. Remember, don't strain after sensations; relax and let them come to you.

Now widen the lens. Hold your whole hand in your attention again, then the whole lower arm, then the whole arm from the shoulder to the fingertips. Finally, hold your whole body in your soft attention. How does the quality of your attention change as you widen your focus? When you hold the whole body in your attention, what happens to the minute particulars of sensation in your fingertip? What happens if you widen the lens to include the sounds in the room and then the distant sounds outside the room?

PRACTICE 1.4
Feel Your Sense Gateways (5–10 minutes)

Seeing, hearing, smelling, tasting, and touching are all embodied experiences to include in your mindfulness practice. In this practice, you consciously feel and relax the sense gateways of your eyes, ears, nose, mouth, and skin.

Sit in a comfortable position and close your eyes. Just as you did with your hand in the previous practice, now bring your attention to the sensation inside your mouth. Sense the touch of your lips against each other, the inner walls of your cheeks, the cave of your palate. Relax the floating mass of your tongue at its root. Empty out any gripping in the jaw and lips. Rest your attention in your mouth long enough to allow the sensation to blossom from virtually unnoticed into lush aliveness.

Is there a taste in your mouth right now? Don't strain to find one— just open to what's there.

Now migrate your attention from your mouth up the inner canal of the left ear, sensing the inner ear, the eardrum, and the intricate shell of the outer ear. Notice whether your eyes have turned to the left, as if trying to *see* your ear. Instead, relax the eyes and sense not the image or idea of your ear but the actual feeling.

Flow your attention through the interior of the head to the right ear and explore it with the same care. Then see what it's like to sense both of your ears simultaneously. Can you do it? Or does your attention flicker back and forth?

Relax the inner ears to receive whatever sounds are present—loud or soft, distant or close. Don't strain to hear them or try to block them out. Include them as part of your meditation, not a distraction from it.

Now flow your attention into the left eye. Sense the upper lid touching the lower lid. Relax all the muscles around the eye. Feel the globe of the eyeball resting in the nest of its socket. Just as you did with the ears, pour your attention from the left to the right eye. Explore it with equal intimacy. Then feel both eyes simultaneously. Relax the backs of the eyes and the optic nerves.

Receive whatever is present in your visual field—which, since your eyes are closed, will probably just be a play of light, color, and darkness. If you'd like, half-open your eyes for a few breaths to receive the dance of form and light all around you. Notice whether your mind immediately starts to manufacture stories about what you are seeing. Instead, just open to the medley of color and shape. Widen your peripheral vision. Then close the eyes again.

With the same relaxed curiosity, travel your attention into your nose. Sense its outer bony structures. Feel your way deep inside to the bright, prickling sensation of air moving through the nostrils and sinuses. Do you feel the breath more vividly in one nostril or the other? Open to whatever smells are present, whether subtle or strong.

Now widen your attention to sense all of your skin, the flexible, tactile organ that covers your whole body. In particular, feel the sensations in the palms of your hands and the soles of your feet. Feel the temperature of the air, the touch of clothes on your body. Soften the skin of your belly and notice the effect on the breath.

Much of your brain is wired up to these organs of sense perception. As they brighten, can you feel your whole being become more sensitive, more alert?

PRACTICE 1.5
Exploring the Whole Body (20–40 minutes)

This body-sensing journey is your core practice for this week—an intimate exploration of the terrain of your own inner world of sensations. It is one variation of the ancient practice of Yoga Nidra—often translated as "yogic sleep"—and of the body-scan technique commonly used in the Buddhist vipassana tradition.

To begin, settle into a comfortable reclining position—flat on your back in Savasana (Corpse Pose). Do whatever you need to make yourself more comfortable: You may wish to drape your knees over a bolster or folded blanket to ease your lower back, or slightly elevate your head on a folded blanket. Cover yourself with a blanket to stay warm. A silk eye pillow can block out light and relax the eyes. Rest for a few breaths and relax into the safety of your environment.

Once you feel at ease, travel your attention through your sense organs, just as you did in the practice 1.4: Feel Your Sense Gateways. Linger in each area—mouth, ears, eyes, and nose—for as long as it takes for that area to blossom into sensation.

From there, move the attention to the skin of the face, then the back of the skull where it makes contact with the ground. Take your time.

With no hurry, travel down into the hollow at the base of your throat. Linger there. Then flow your attention like honey down through your body.

It doesn't matter what route you take. One pathway is to journey from the throat to the heart; then down the bones of first one arm, then the other; then linger while feeling both hands simultaneously. From there return to the heart and move slowly down to the belly, pelvis, and reproductive organs. Then travel down one leg to the foot, then down the other, then rest in both feet at the same time.

The pathway is not important. The quality of intimacy and connection you bring to the exploration is what matters—plus the emphasis on feeling the sensation from the inside rather than visualizing the body part you're exploring.

Bring playfulness to this investigation. Some days you may want to travel very slowly, diving deeply into the intricacies of, say, the hand—feeling each finger individually or each joint of a finger or each half of a joint of a finger. Other days you may want to hold a broader lens. Don't strain to locate or magnify sensations. Just relax and allow them to emerge.

Some areas of your body may feel dead, numb, or invisible. That's fine. Trust that your body will talk to you in its own way, in its own right time. What you are doing now is creating a safe space in which that conversation can occur.

Just as with any meditation, as you do this practice, your attention will inevitably drift away, and you will find yourself wandering the aisles of a candy store of thinking (or, perhaps, wandering in a hell realm of your own creation). When you notice that this has happened, just bring yourself back to the last body part you remember being present for. Reconnect with feeling and gently resume your explorations. If you find yourself repeatedly drifting away at the same body part, just notice this tendency. Don't spin stories around it.

When you have completed your leisurely journey, widen your focus to hold your whole body. Sense yourself as infinite sky dotted with flickering stars of sensation arising and passing away.

A note on the audio download: It's lovely to be guided through this practice, as you can be guided in the downloadable video for this week. But be sure to practice it on your own as well. That way you'll learn important lessons about how and why you drift away from awareness when you're not being continually prompted from the outside to return.

Each time you carry the flashlight of your focused awareness through the darkened corridors of your body, its beam will get brighter, and more and more of your inner experience will be illuminated. Locked rooms will open, yielding treasure troves of sensation.

Try this: Practice this body scan in any position. Try it in a supported restorative yoga pose such as Supta Baddha Konasana (Reclining Bound Angle Pose) or in a simple standing pose like Tadasana (Mountain Pose).

In Your Asana This Week

All of the practices we have explored this week are wonderful ways to begin a session of asana or pranayama. From one of the body-sensing practices, flow into your movement or breath work with deepened sensitivity. Can you stay connected to the area that you were exploring in stillness as you move and breathe? Can you shift the lens of your focus to other areas—say, the alignment of the shoulder joint in Downward Dog—and feel that part of your body come alive in the same way? Can you open to the breath as living sensation?

In Your Seated Meditation Practice This Week

Be sure to leave at least 10 to 15 minutes at the end of your practice time for seated meditation—you will gradually increase this as the program progresses. In week 5 there is more detail about the specifics of the seated-meditation posture. For now, just pick any seated posture in which you can be both comfortable and alert and in which the spine can be both upright and relaxed. Don't feel that you need to sit cross-legged on the floor; it's fine to use a chair if that's more comfortable for you.

Meditators are often instructed to focus on the breath as the anchor for their attention. But if you aren't solidly grounded in the felt sense of the body, the breath can feel like an abstract concept rather than a vibrant, living sensation. For that reason, in your seated meditation practice this week, begin by using your body sensations as the anchor for your attention, just as you've been doing in your other practices. You'll train your capacity for sustained presence by bringing your mind back—again and again—into some aspect of your present embodied experience.

Once you've settled into your sitting posture, invite your attention to flow through your body just as you did in the reclining version, Exploring the Whole Body. For consistency, it's nice to follow the same pathway that you followed while reclining—beginning with the sense organs, then journeying on. Notice what it's like to let your attention travel through your body when seated. Is it easier or more difficult for you than doing it while lying down? Some people find it easier to stay alert and focused while sitting. Other people find that the seated posture makes it more difficult for them to relax and connect with subtle feelings.

Once you've completed a leisurely pass through the body, you have a choice about where to focus your "lens of awareness."

- Continue to cycle your attention through the body. With every pass through, let your exploration become deeper and more sensitive.
- Ground your attention in some specific part of your body and return to the felt sense of that touch point again and again—the hands, for instance, or the feet.
- Widen the lens of your awareness to hold the whole body simultaneously, as you did at the conclusion of your reclining body scan. Rest in the wave of breath coming and going as a whole-body sensation. Sense yourself as the space in which the breath waves arise and pass.
- If you felt the breath most strongly in one particular area—say, the belly, the chest, or the opening of the nostrils—let your attention rest in the sensation in this area.

Be clear what your choice is and use it as your anchor. Inevitably, whatever approach you choose, another one will start to seem more appealing halfway through your meditation. Avoid dithering. Stay with the one you've chosen. Reassure yourself that in your very next meditation, you will be able to pick another one.

Repeatedly drawing the attention back to a specific aspect of your physical experience is a form of concentration (*samatha*) practice; it's designed to gather the fragmented heart and mind, nourishing a sense of stability and ease. However, it's perfectly normal for it to illuminate, first of all, just how scattered you really are. No matter what anchor point you've chosen, you'll inevitably drift off entirely. You won't just be fantasizing about other meditation approaches. You'll be fantasizing about whole other lives. When you find that happening, don't beat yourself up. Give your fantasy self a hug and then tell her: not now. Right now we're listening to the body as it comes to us with all the feelings we've been too busy to hear.

In Your Daily Life This Week

Set a timer on your phone or computer to chime at certain times throughout the day or at regular intervals. When you hear the bell, pause and connect with an anchor point that works for you—your hands, perhaps, or the soles of your feet. Give yourself a minute or two to feel sensation blossom there.

If it's appropriate, you can close your eyes—but it's also great to practice this without stopping your activities. Sense your hands while you're doing dishes or tapping on the computer or digging in the garden. Feel your feet while you're walking or driving. Notice whether it's possible to continue to feel your body while shopping, while talking on the phone, while sending an e-mail. When is it easy for you to connect with the felt sense of your body? When is it difficult?

RESOURCES

For continuing to explore the kind of intimate, relaxed body-sensing practice that we've been doing this week, I can't think of a better resource than Richard Miller's yoga nidra books, CDs, and downloadable practices. You can get them all at www.irest.us. I learned yoga nidra from him and continue to be inspired by the depth of his practice and service. Frank Jude Boccio's excellent book *Mindfulness Yoga* is a great resource for grounding your mindful yoga practice in yogic and Buddhist philosophy.

Exploring Your Body in Action

FOR CHRISTMAS a few years ago, my partner, Teja, gave me a round yoga mat about six feet in diameter. When I spread it out and began to practice—by the twinkle of the Christmas tree lights—I was amazed at the way my asanas transformed. My gestures became rounder, less angular. I took up more space. I spiraled and spun. To my astonishment, I realized that my thirty years of yoga practice had been unconsciously shaped by the boxy confines of a 6-by-2½-foot rubber rectangle.

There's nothing wrong with a rectangular mat, of course. They're useful and practical tools. And a circular mat would reveal its own limitations in time: Why am I not flowing through the whole room? Why am I not flinging open the windows and doors and dancing through them?

A yoga mat is only one way we may unconsciously box in our journey of awakening by outside forms. The yoga poses themselves, when practiced rigidly or unconsciously, can become constraints on our freedom rather than means for unfolding. A meditation practice can become just one more way to try to establish ourselves as the supreme dictator over our inner world—and then beat ourselves up when we don't succeed.

So this week we're going to explore ways to stay awake in our bodies while moving in and through and around the forms of yoga asanas. We're going to build on the sensitivity to our inner landscape that we cultivated in our first week of practice by extending it into conscious movement—with an emphasis not on *what* we are doing in our yoga practice but *how much we feel* as we are doing it. We'll continue our exploration of the lens of our attention as we learn to make choices about where we place our awareness as we move—as well as learning more about how our attention naturally flows in response to our ever-changing activities. And we'll deepen our visceral understanding that awareness is vaster than all of the sensations and movements that arise and pass away inside it.

Also this week, as we explore our physical bodies through conscious movement, we'll learn to flow skillfully between three important dimensions of our practice: meeting and accepting our bodies exactly as they are; skillfully working to free them of limiting habitual patterns of contraction; and cultivating positive qualities of energy, openness, and sensitivity. These three foundational aspects of mindful practice will show up again and again at every stage of our exploration together, whether we're working with our physical bodies, our breath, our hearts, or our minds.

■ For a guided practice based on the principles in week 2, go to annecushman.com/practices.

THE ART OF EXPLORATION

To begin, here's something to remember about yoga poses: people made them up.

Some of them were made up a long time ago—hundreds or even thousands of years. A lot of them—including many that we think of today as "classic" yoga poses—were invented by Indian yogis in the early part of the twentieth century. Some were imported from places as diverse as YMCA exercise classes and Swedish gymnastics and then given Sanskrit names. Some were invented as recently as last week. There is nothing inherently sacred about any of the postures that you'll see arcing and twisting on yoga calendars. What makes them sacred is the way we inhabit them.

There are really only so many ways the human body can move, and people in different cultures and different eras have probed those limits. It seems likely that the earliest forms of asana practice were spontaneous eruptions from deep meditative states, the trembling of psycho-spiritual energy throughout the body releasing into movement. Then hatha yogis began imitating and systematizing those spontaneous movements in order to access the states that had originally inspired them.

I don't say this to denigrate the formal yoga asanas we commonly practice today, which are powerful tools for transformation that shape the body and the psyche over a lifetime of practice. They are an extraordinary expression of the possibilities of the human body, a conduit for energy, and a vehicle for exploring our inner world. Yoga poses can be precisely honed instruments for addressing structural imbalances that may be reflecting, perpetuating, or even creating imbalances in the mind. And tuning in to the nuances of somatic experience is a compelling way to harness the attention. So attending to the principles of postural alignment is one important aspect of a mindful yoga practice.

But what we think of as a "pose" is just a moment of flow frozen in a snapshot. It's no more or less significant than the moment that came right before it. Snapshots are evocative ways to perpetuate memories: You're glad you have that photo of you and your best friend toasting your birthday in the cabin in Yosemite. But the photo doesn't show what happened a few minutes later, when a black bear broke in and took the whole door off its hinges.

So in your practice this week, let go of any fixation on form so you can really feel your body moving from the inside. Sensations are the language of the body. Listen to your own body's story as if hearing a friend confide secrets she's never shared before. Tune in to the parts of your body that are crying out to be heard—and also to those areas that may have been numbed into silence.

Move from feeling—and allow your movements, in turn, to bring more feeling to areas that may be invisible to your awareness. Open locked rooms, explore hidden crannies, fling open the shutters in airless garrets. Let alignment arise organically out of your body's innate intelligence.

Practice your yoga as a way of opening the boxes you have put yourself inside, not jamming yourself into more of them. What other shapes have you forced yourself to assume in your life? Where else might your perception of how freely you can move be constrained by other people's conventions?

Along the way, you'll discover parts of your body that are stuck, injured, or vulnerable. Be with them with particular tenderness, not as obstacles to success but as gifts to be unwrapped. Ask them how they want to be healed or released. By being with yourself in this way, you are expanding your capacity to attend your inner world with kindness and sensitivity—a capacity that will serve you well as you turn your attention to more and more subtle aspects of your experience.

Remember, it's not just structures and alignment that you are feeling into. Yes, you are tuning in to your proprioception of bones and organs and muscles and skin and their optimum relationship and function. But as you go deeper, such anatomical distinctions begin to dissolve. Your body emerges in your awareness as a shimmering field of sensations—appearing and disappearing like bats swooping under a street lamp. What you think of as *hand* breaks down into a pixelated field of dancing detail, just as an impressionist's painting of a lake is composed of thousands of tiny dots of color.

Use the conventions of the yoga asanas as chisels to open your range of movement, build your strength, and awaken your body's intelligence. But then move through them and beyond them. They are a trail map helping you navigate a majestic wilderness. But don't confuse them with the silver river flowing between granite cliffs or the red-tailed hawk soaring over them, clutching a fish in its talons.

Don't just tramp down the well-traveled fire roads of a familiar pose. Instead, meander down all the deer trails. Stop at a hidden beach for a picnic. Sit on the sand and listen to seagulls call, and take a bite of an apple you pluck off an overhanging branch—sweet and crisp and tasting of rain and eternity.

Go Slowly to Feel More

When cultivating this art of moving from your inner impulse, it's useful, especially at first, to move at a leisurely pace.

You can be vibrantly alive while flowing through an intense vinyasa practice or running up a mountain trail, cold rain stinging your cheeks. One sect of Korean Zen monks does outdoor running meditation, thundering through the fields around the monastery with their robes flapping.

But for most of us, it's easier to build our capacity to be present if we're moving slowly, at least at first. How slow should you go? My favorite qigong teacher puts it like this: *Go no faster than you can stay connected to feeling.*

On a mindfulness meditation retreat, you might do an eating meditation in which you take ten minutes to eat a single raisin: turning it in your fingers to feel its shriveled surface, holding it up to your nose to smell its spicy sweetness, chewing it to mush and feeling the deft movements of your tongue against your teeth as flavor floods your taste buds.

It can be useful to slow down your asana practice to a similar pace. When you slow down, you have a greater chance of being able to drop below your concepts about something—whether it's a cucumber or a Downward Dog—and into the living experience. In your yoga practice, you have the chance to notice habitual holdings and movements—the part of your spine that doesn't bend and the part that overbends, the way you reflexively place your feet a certain distance apart. You may notice that you've been forcing yourself into some poses in a way that is stressing your knee or lower back, or have been holding back in other poses through unacknowledged fears.

You may see aspects of your practice that you have been performing habitually for years—and perhaps even teaching to others—that no longer serve you. And you'll cultivate a direct knowledge of your inner world that allows you to trust your own impulses rather than reflexively following the dictates of other people.

Does Mindful Yoga Have to Be Slow?

Mindful yoga involves making intelligent choices about how to practice so that our practice responds appropriately to the needs of the situation in which we find ourselves. And there are many times when a vigorous, fast-paced practice is exactly what's needed. Here are just a few such situations:

- You are buzzing with excess energy that needs to be channeled or released.

- Your energy feels sluggish, stagnant, sleepy. You may not feel like moving, but if you tried to sit in meditation or do restorative poses, you'd drop off to sleep.
- Your body is stressed and tense from a long day at work, sitting at the computer or around conference tables under fluorescent lights. You just need to sweat, flow, breathe, and feel good—maybe with some music cranked up.
- You simply need a good workout—and yoga is your exercise of choice.

A good teacher wouldn't offer the identical practice to elderly people in a nursing home, at-risk teenagers, and pregnant women. Assess your own situation and give yourself the practices that are most needed—at the pace that they are needed—to bring about a state of relaxed, alert presence.

But be sure that you're not simply reverting to your unexamined belief systems about the "right" way to practice. Experiment with different paces—including slowing a familiar practice way down—so you can know from the inside how each affects your body, nervous system, heart, and mind.

THE ART OF LONG HOLDS

Another useful tool for awakening to sensation is to settle into a chosen pose for an extended period of time so that deeper and deeper layers of your body and psyche can begin to reveal themselves.

When you hold a yoga asana for an extended period, you are not just breezing in and out of your body for a quick "Hi, how's it going?" (You know how those conversations go—the only acceptable answer, really, is "Pretty good. How about you?") Instead, you're settling down to spend some quality time with a good friend. You're asking as if you really want to know: "How *are* you?" Then you're sticking around to hear the answer, even if it takes awhile.

This is a different mode of practice from spontaneous, moving exploration. Here, you are consciously submitting yourself to specific limitations of structure and time to see what that reveals. As one Zen saying goes: *Put a snake in a bamboo pole and it discovers its true nature.*

A yin yoga practice is a wonderful tool for this kind of exploration. In yin yoga, we put our body in long-held passive poses that put pressure on the muscles, the connective tissues, and the subtle energy channels that flow through them. On the physical level, yin yoga allows the deeper layers of the body—the denser, tighter tissues of ligaments and connective tissues—to release in a way that they don't have time to do when we are moving more quickly. In the subtle body, yin yoga is said to stimulate the life force—the prana or qi—to move through the energy pathways and nourish the ligaments and joints.

A yin yoga practice is a great way to prepare the body for seated meditation—among other benefits, it opens the hips and maintains flexibility in the sacro-lumbar joint. But it's also a meditation in itself, in which your arising experience percolates through the filter of your sustained attention. As the deep tissues of the body let go, they release memories, emotions, and dreams. As you rest in the yin poses, you attune your inner ears to a symphony played by your whole being.

It's also good to explore long holds in dynamic postures—such as standing poses like Triangle and Warrior—although you will probably not be able to stay with them for as long. Don't look at this as an endurance test or get rigid in order to stay in the pose longer. Instead, think of "holding" the pose as if you were holding a baby in your arms.

When you practice long holds of dynamic poses, you encourage both persistence and relaxation—the ability to stay with a challenging task in a gentle but steady way over a sustained period. So many things in life require this kind of fluid persistence: launching a company, raising a child, recording a song, saving a rain forest. So it's good to have a place to practice it where the stakes aren't so terribly high.

STAYING GROUNDED   Annie Mahon

Annie Mahon is the director of the Circle Yoga Center in Washington, D.C.

Yoga practice really helped mindfulness practice become part of who I am, not just another thing to talk about at dinner.

My daughter went through some really hard times when she was in college. I had to go there to help her deal with the police. I know that if I had not been able to be present with her and stay grounded in my body, I would have gone off the deep end. Instead, I was able to go with her where she needed to go emotionally and help her decide what to do. When I reflect back, that time doesn't feel like a crisis. It feels like "Oh, it was really hard, but I was there for it." It was very unpleasant for everyone, but it doesn't feel like it left the kind of scar it would have left if I had been lost in anxiety and panic.

WEEK 2 PRACTICES

This week, start every practice session with last week's Arriving in Your Body (page 38) or Exploring the Whole Body (page 44). Then choose whether you want the day's asana practice to focus more on movement exploration, more on developing your capacity for sustained attention through long holds of one asana at a time, or more on opening a conversation with parts of your body that are harder to access. Here are some sample sequences:

Day 1, movement exploration: Start with Feeling the Hands in Movement (below), Feeling the Arms in Movement (page 60), Exploring the Body in Movement (page 61), and The Journey of Downward Dog (page 62). Then go on to explore other poses in that free-form fashion, lingering at least 5 minutes in each pose.

Day 2, movement exploration: Explore Shifting the Lens of Awareness in Movement (page 64) in Half Sun Salutations, and then continue that practice through a variety of vinyasa flows—a good way to get in a more vigorous workout while continuing to train your mindful presence.

Day 3, long holds: Go from your initial check-in straight to Long Hold of a Yin Pose (page 67). Then do a whole yin sequence of anywhere from 30 to 90 minutes, holding each pose for 4 to 8 minutes.

Day 4, long holds: For a more strength-oriented practice, begin with Long Hold of a Standing Posture (page 69), followed by a 30- to 40-minute sequence of standing postures that you hold for 3 to 5 minutes apiece.

Day 5, opening what's stuck: After your initial check-in, focus on contacting areas of your body that are harder for you to feel by going directly to the practice of Opening What's Stuck or Numb (page 70).

Days 6–7: Now that you've explored different approaches to practice, choose whatever combination best meets your practice needs this day.

After each asana session, be sure to leave at least 15 minutes for seated meditation (this week's instructions are on page 71). Notice how your deepening relationship with your body is affecting your sitting practice.

PRACTICE 2.6

Feeling the Hands in Movement (2–3 minutes)

In this practice you'll apply the ability to sense your body in stillness that you cultivated last week and sustain it through simple, exploratory movement. It's easy to feel your body when you're creating strong sensations through vigorous movement. Here, you're cultivating the more subtle art of maintaining intimate presence throughout a routine action.

Come to a comfortable seated position with your hands in your lap, palms facing up. Just as you did in last week's exercise, Feel Both Hands (page 41), guide your attention to rest in the felt sense of your hands.

After your hands light up in your awareness, slowly begin to curl the fingers of both hands into a tight fist. Notice what the movement does to the sensations. You may feel an explosion of feeling. Or you may find that as you start to move, your attention fades and diffuses. Either way, stay present with the sensations as they change. When your hands are fully folded shut, pause for a moment, then begin to gradually unfurl the fingers until the hands have blossomed all the way open. Then pause again for a heartbeat.

Continue to slowly close and open the hands. Do you feel them most precisely when they are fully closed or opened? Or during the transitions? Where does your attention drift off? What happens to your breath as the hands open and close?

When you have finished, pause and sense your hands in stillness.

PRACTICE 2.7
Feeling the Arms in Movement (3–5 minutes)

Raising and lowering the arms is a gesture you do over and over in yoga, so it's easy to go on autopilot. Here, notice what it's like to deepen into a familiar gesture, advancing your practice not through increased physical complexity but through heightened sensitivity.

Begin as you did in the previous practice of Feeling the Hands in Movement. This time, after furling and unfurling the hands a few times, allow the opening in the hands to flow up the arms so that the arms begin to lift away from the sides of the body and float up. Pulse them a few times—dropping them down and opening them away from the body again—letting the movement get a little larger each time. The arms can reach to the sides and overhead, or they can float up in front of you, or they can open out sideways as if in an embrace; the precise gesture doesn't matter. What's important is how intimately you connect with the gesture of opening and closing. Where in your body do you sense the movement originating? What happens to your breath as the arms raise and lower?

Notice the pathways that your attention travels when you keep the arms moving in a more structured, linear way—up and down to the sides or front, for example. Then begin to break the movement up into free-form spirals, a playful exploration of nonlinear space. Let the arms billow like seaweed on ocean waves. How does the quality of your sensate attention change? Where does your attention most easily gather: in the area of strongest sensation? The area of greatest movement?

What is this thing we call "attention" that migrates here and there, sometimes flowing on its own and sometimes under our direction? Who is paying attention? Who is running the show?

PRACTICE 2.8
Exploring the Body in Movement—Cat-Cow (5 minutes)

Our energy flows where we place our attention. By learning the art of directing your attention—without forcing it—while in motion, you are cultivating a powerful tool for presence and healing that you can carry into your life and relationships.

Kneel on your hands and knees, palms under your shoulders and knees under your hips. Before you begin to move, sense into the weight and density of your bones. Connect with the wind of your breath blowing through the forest of your organs, bones, and skin.

Begin simple Cat-Cow rolls, initiating the movement from the tailbone. Tuck the tailbone under and let the movement ripple up the spine until it reaches the head, the belly drawing back and the spine rounded. Then, from the tip of the tailbone, let the movement ripple in the other direction. Imagine your spine as an undulating snake, with its head at your tailbone.

Physically, this is a simple gesture. So as you move, let your challenge be this: How much can you feel? Can you give yourself the gift of your own rapt attention?

For a few repetitions, notice where the lens of your attention naturally focuses: The area that is moving the most? The area of strongest sensation? Do you hold the whole body in a broad, soft lens, or do you dial in on a particular location? Does that location stay the same, or does your attention travel from one place to another?

Then, for a few rounds, focus your attention in the spine. With every undulation call your attention deeper and deeper inside the muscles around the spine, the vertebrae, the spinal cord. As you hold the spine in the foreground of your attention, how much of your awareness still holds the larger field of your body? How much remains in the hands, the feet, the skin?

Now let the movement open up into playful exploration. Draw circles in the air with your tailbone. Bend the arms so the chest dips toward the floor, then away, as you continue to glide. Again, notice where your attention travels. Broaden your lens and watch the sparks of sensation fly up from the bonfire of your movement. Then dial it in more precisely: the tip of the tailbone, the pressure of the roots of the fingers into the ground, the space between the vertebrae. Can you continue to flow and breathe as your focus narrows?

There are no right answers to these questions. You are engaged in an ever-deepening relationship with the nature of sensation.

When you have completed your exploration, settle back into Child's Pose. Notice where your attention lands. Notice how, even within stillness, movement continues.

Try this: Practice this kind of exploration in any repetitive, oscillating movement. Flowing from Downward Dog to Upward Dog. Bending the knee in and out of a lunge or Warrior Pose. Try some of these variations or any others that occur to you. As the poses get more physically challenging, does your ability to track sensation increase or decrease? Some people find that stronger sensations are easier to feel. Other people find that despite their best efforts, they begin to put their emphasis more on the execution of the pose and less on the inner sensing.

PRACTICE 2.9
The Journey of Downward Dog (5 minutes)

Here we'll explore playing within and around the form of a familiar pose, with an eye to awakening the flow of aliveness. For simplicity's sake, let's do it with Downward Dog, that favorite yoga standby, but this kind of exploration can be done in any pose. If it's difficult for you to support your weight in Downward Dog, you can do this same exploration with your hands pressing into the wall or resting on the edge of a chair.

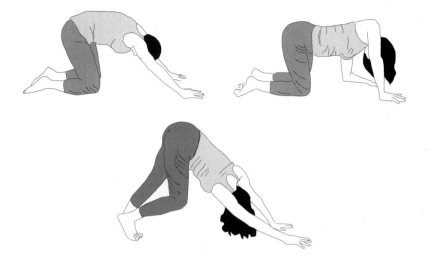

Begin on all fours, as in Cat-Cow. Root your hands, inviting in the sense of connection with the earth. Roll your spine a few times as in Cat-Cow. Then gradually begin to lift your pelvis toward the sky, as if it were being buoyed up by a balloon inside your belly. Come to full extension slowly over the course of several breaths. Notice whether you view the journey into the pose as less worthy of your attention than the destination. At what point do you consider that you have "arrived"?

Once you consider yourself "there," rest for a few breaths in what you have labeled "Downward Dog." Then begin to liquefy the pose into movement. Move slowly, letting the movement originate from deep in your belly and ripple outward. Bend first one knee, then the other, allowing the hip to drop and the thighbone to swing loosely. Lift a leg high and open the hip joint, rolling the belly open, then draw spirals with the femur. Ripple the spine in waves from the tail to the crown of the head. Notice the sensations that blossom as you do. Don't hairspray the pose—let it blow in the wind of your breath.

Let a yoga pose become like a trellis that you twine over and around and through before you burst into bloom. In a garden, a grapevine reaches off its lattice and grabs on to a nearby tomato plant. A squash sends exploratory tendrils across the ground. Do you want to be the trellis? Or do you want to be the living, fruiting vine?

Hold the moving, breathing shape in a wide lens. Where are the strongest areas of sensation, and what are they? Tingling? Pulsing? Heat? Throbbing? Notice whether you are labeling the sensation anatomically: *Shoulder. Hip. Neck.* Then drop below the label into the sensation itself.

Periodically pause in stillness, finding the organic alignment of the skeleton that best supports and expresses a sense of balance and ease. What you think of as the pose may or may not be the most balanced and restful place to pause. Now scan through your body and see if there are any unnecessary areas of gripping—jaw, eyes, belly, pelvic floor. When you release extra gripping, does it affect your ability to feel elsewhere in the body?

You will come across areas that feel contracted or frozen, that don't move in the way your mind may want them to. Greet these places with kindness: *Hello, grumpy hip. Hello, tight shoulder. Hello, stuck vertebrae.* Notice any tendency to think of these places as a problem that you must rush to fix. Instead, hang out with them awhile as they are. What do they feel like? What are they asking from you? Developing this capacity to accept and investigate parts of yourself—without immediately imposing an agenda for transformation—is central to the art of mindfulness.

Continue this exploration for at least 5 minutes. If your arms get tired, feel free to come in and out of the pose a few times. In between, rest in Child's Pose and notice what happens to the quality of your attention. Are you able to be equally present at times that you label the "in between" or "after" periods? If the impulse arises to "get on to the next pose, already!" notice where you feel that impulse in your body. Then use it as a springboard to dive even deeper into your experience of this moment.

Try this: Do this same type of exploration in any pose with which you are relatively at ease. Be sure to stay well back from your edge so you have "wiggle room." What happens to your ability to experiment within and around a shape as the shapes get more challenging?

PRACTICE 2.10

Shifting the Lens of Awareness in Movement— Half Sun Salutations (15 minutes)

We can deepen our exploration of shifting the lens of our attention—just as we did in Focus the Lens of Awareness (practice 1.3wC on page 42)—

by exploring the conscious shifting of attention while flowing through movement.

For simplicity's sake, we'll use a sequence that is familiar to most yoga practitioners—the Half Sun Salutation.

As a yoga practitioner, you are already skilled at placing your attention in a specific area in order to make some precise adjustment. Here we are going to use that finely honed skill in the service of pure, receptive attention—while in motion.

Begin by coming into standing position in balanced alignment. Then, just as you did in the Feeling the Hands in Movement practice (page 59), rest your attention in your hands. Let them come alive to you. Invite about 70 percent of your attention into your hands while the other 30 percent of your attention holds the whole field of your body and breath.

Now begin to flow through your Half Sun Salutations, moving slowly. Keep the hands in the foreground of your awareness, letting the rest of your body and breath recede into the background—as if your hands were playing a solo in the orchestra of your body sensations while the rest of the body is playing an accompaniment.

After a few rounds of Half Sun Salutations, release your attention out of your hands as you come into standing. Seamlessly draw your attention into your feet instead and continue the Half Sun Salutations as the feet now play their solo. If it helps to maintain your focus, you can make a soft mental note to yourself as you flow: *Feet. Feet. Feet.*

Continue this process for multiple rounds of Half Sun Salutations, moving your attention in turn to various body parts. I often work with the following sequence: hands, feet, third eye (directly above and between the eyebrows), throat, heart, belly, pelvic floor. But you can also focus on other areas, such as the tip of the tailbone, the base of the skull, the root of the tongue, the jaw, or the shoulders.

Discover what areas are difficult for you to contact as you move and breathe, and which are easy. Notice, too, the quality with which you invite an area to come to the foreground. Do you jerk or strain your attention? Do other parts of your body tense in the effort to focus?

For your last few rounds, open your lens wide. Listen to the symphony of all of those body parts singing together. Discover what voices naturally come to the foreground. Then rest in stillness in standing and notice what you feel.

Try this: Practice this shifting of the lens with any repetitive sequence, even long ones—different variations of full Sun Salutations, for example, or with any other vinyasa flow that you know well. Notice what happens to your ability to guide your attention as the sequences become more complex and physically demanding. Is your attention drawn reflexively to the areas of strongest sensation or to the familiar adjustments of alignment?

Or try setting a timer to chime every 5 minutes as you flow through your regular yoga practice, whatever that is—a strong Ashtanga series, a gentle Kripalu flow, a hot Bikram workout. Every time the timer pings, shift your focus to a new area. When do you slip back into autopilot? What is it like to keep your attention moving in an unfamiliar way while following a familiar pattern?

PRACTICE 2.11
Holding a Steady Anchor (15–30 minutes)

This practice is almost the inverse of practice 2.10, Shifting the Lens of Awareness in Movement. Instead of regularly shifting your focal point, you will pick one steady anchor for your attention and hold it for your entire practice period. Like practice 2.10, it can be done in any asana sequence.

Choose one simple but precise detail of your physical experience to serve as your anchor. Examples include (but are not limited to)

- the triangles formed on the soles of your feet by the heel, the ball of the big toe, and the ball of the little toe;
- the soft center of the palm of your hand, surrounded by the pressure points of the base of the fingers;
- the relationship between the domes of the pelvic floor, the diaphragm, and the soft palate;
- the tender spot just below the occipital bone, where the base of the skull meets the neck;
- the hinge of the jaw and the root of the tongue;

- the space between the pubic bone and the sternum and the corresponding area on the back of the body.

As you move through your practice, return to your chosen anchor again and again, in pose after pose. Does it feel different in different postures? Sometimes it will feel central to a pose; other times it will be more peripheral. How does that affect the quality of attention you are able to give it? Notice how it fades in and out of the foreground of your awareness.

When you have finished your practice, let go of your deliberate focus on your anchor and rest in Savasana with the lens of your attention wide open.

PRACTICE 2.12
Long Hold of a Yin Pose (3–5 minutes)

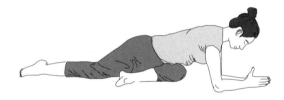

In this practice we're going to hold a yin yoga posture for an extended period as a somatic meditation. Remember, a yin yoga pose is a posture that you can sustain for an extended period of time in a relaxed way without muscular engagement but that places sufficient pressure on your tissues to create a strong sensation. A good choice for this practice might be a Pigeon Pose (pictured here; often known as Sleeping Swan in the yin yoga style), the Sphinx Pose, or a Wide-Legged Forward Bend—but you can choose any other yin posture or sequence of postures with which you are familiar. (See the resources section on page 72 for where to get more information about yin yoga practice.)

I recommend 3- to 5-minute holds (on each side) to begin, using a timer to ensure consistency. As your physical capacities and ability to stay present increase, you can gradually increase the length of time to whatever feels workable for you.

Set yourself up in the chosen posture with attention to safe alignment, staying well back from your physical edge. You are not charging into the pose as if invading a small country, overpowering it with your shock-and-awe yoga tactics. Instead, when you meet resistance, pause until you are invited in more deeply.

You may feel strong sensations in the muscle tissues, but if you feel a sharp pain in a joint, back off. If the sensation becomes so uncomfortable that your body begins to tense, your breath grows ragged, or you are not able to be present in a relaxed way, then back off until the sensation becomes more manageable. Your intention is not to stretch your physical limits but to cultivate your ability to feel.

Once you have established the basic shape of the pose, let your attention settle into the felt sense of your body. Begin with a wide lens for 5 to 10 breaths, holding the whole body in your attention. Then notice what area is calling to you through strong sensation. Maybe it's your outer hip, burning and tingling. Maybe it's a sense of warmth and pressure across your lower back. Maybe it's the movement of your body in response to the breath. Gradually let your attention start to magnetize toward that area. Let about 70 percent of your attention collect in that area of strong sensation.

Then begin to explore its nature. Let go of any beliefs or concepts about anatomical structures—"hips" or "shoulders" or "knees"—and rest in the pure sensations. What does it feel like from the inside? Do you feel heat? Pressure? Tingling? Burning? Does the feeling have a texture or a color? Does the sensation stay constant, or does it pulse and throb? Does it stay in one place, or does it move around?

Pay attention not just to the sensation but to the attitude with which you are meeting it. Are you grasping at the sensation? Pushing it away? Are you meeting it with friendship, or do you subtly or not so subtly judge it and wish to control it?

If your attention drifts off to thinking about your experience, guide it back to feeling from the inside.

If the area of strong sensation shifts location, let your attention follow it. Observe what percentage of your attention stays with the area of strong sensation and what percentage attends to other aspects of your experience—other sensations in your body or the movement of your breath. Encourage the area of strongest sensation to remain in the foreground.

At the end of your exploration, widen the lens again to sense the whole body for a few breaths before releasing from the pose. If you are practicing an asymmetrical posture, take the pose on the other side, seeing how present you can be throughout the transition.

PRACTICE 2.13
Long Hold of a Standing Posture (3–5 minutes)

In this practice we explore sensation while holding a dynamic pose. Long holds of dynamic postures are an especially satisfying way to practice if you're used to a rigorous physical asana workout and are feeling resistant to the slow explorations we've been doing. This way you can cultivate mindful presence while still working your body strongly.

Long holds can be practiced with any dynamic pose that you can hold for several minutes without strain. Set a timer for 3 minutes to begin with, then gradually increase the time to 5 minutes or more.

To start, I suggest a vigorous but stable posture such as Warrior I, Warrior II, or Side Angle Pose. Don't immediately drop into your full version of the pose—instead, move to an edge that you feel confident you can sustain.

Don't think of "holding" the pose as locking the joints and gripping the muscles, although of course there will be muscular activity. Instead, hold with relaxed strength. Let the pose pulse with the breath. Instead of turning away from the area of strongest sensation, turn toward it. If muscles start to burn, walk into the fire with curiosity.

As you tire, continue to hold not by gripping the outer musculature but by relaxing it. Learn to hold from a deeper place—as if your energy body could support your physical form. Notice whether you're enlisting body parts in your war effort that aren't serving you—gripping your jaw, for example, or tensing your belly. If your arms start to ache, instead of tensing your neck muscles, can you relax them?

To hold a dynamic standing pose in this way, your energy needs to drop out of your head and deep into your belly and legs. You don't want to be the kind of warrior who dominates and invades. You want to be the warrior who stands up for justice, who speaks truth in the face of lies.

If you are struggling to hold the pose past your capacity to be present for sensation, back off. If you need to come out before the bell goes off, please do. You want to entrain kindness and relaxed persistence into your nervous system—not harshness and contraction.

If you find yourself habitually coming out early, then set the timer for a shorter period. Be realistic, but give yourself some structure. This is a skillful use of form—as something to surrender into and learn from, like that snake in the bamboo pole.

Try this: Practice these long holds with several of your favorite dynamic poses. Then try them with several of your least-favorite dynamic poses. What difference do you notice?

PRACTICE 2.14
Opening What's Stuck or Numb (45 minutes)

This practice is lovely as a follow-up to an in-depth practice of Exploring the Whole Body (page 44).

First, lie in a comfortable position and do the Exploring the Whole Body practice. If you've been practicing it regularly, you'll find that you'll be able to move your attention through the body in 5 to 10 minutes. Notice the areas that are most difficult for you to feel.

Choose one of these areas and let it know that you are there for it and that you understand that it has good reasons for being shut down. *Hello, upper back. You're feeling tight today. That's okay. I understand why you might not want to open.* Tell it you're there to help, not to push. *Hello, hip. What might help you feel safe enough to release?*

Then—with compassionate curiosity—begin to move into yoga asanas that specifically bring movement or sensation into that area. For example, if your belly is hard to access, you might practice Reclining Butterfly or a supported Bridge Pose. If the heart area feels contracted, try a gentle Cobra or Camel Pose or a restorative back bend over a bolster. If the breath isn't moving in the back body, take a relaxed forward bend, Child's Pose, or Wide-Legged Forward Bend and invite the breath to spread into the kidneys and back ribs. If you can't feel your pelvic floor, gently engage and release Mula Bandha a few times; hold a relaxed Happy Baby Pose, breathing into the area between the sitting bones; or move the energy into the lower body through some hip openers such as Gomukhasana. Bring fluidity to a rigid spine by oscillating through some Cat-Cows or Downward Dog–Upward Dog flows. If your jaw is locked, try a few rounds of Lion's Breath, or simply exhale through the mouth with a soft *ahhhh* sound.

Discover for yourself when it is most effective to open an area through movement and when it is most effective to employ sustained holds. Remember that your intention here is not so much to open the area physically or "improve" your body (although with practice, physical opening will occur); rather, your intention is to increase your ability to feel that part of your body from the inside.

Remember this basic principle: Feeling flows best within a relaxed body. That doesn't mean that there can't be muscular effort involved. It just means that the muscular activity should have a quality of ease about it. If you push into a pose, you may in fact experience heightened sensation while you are in it. But that does nothing for your ability to open to the subtle sensations and emotions that inhabit that region of your body when you are not exerting it.

As you do these poses, don't try to force sensation to arise or get discouraged if it doesn't. You are creating a safe space into which your body can begin to speak—sometimes voicing feelings that have been shut down for years. So don't be the torturer trying to beat a confession out of a silent body part. Be the good friend, patient and present for as long as it takes for your body to confide its secrets.

In Your Seated Meditation Practice This Week

After doing your movement-meditation exploration each day, be sure to save at least 15 minutes for seated meditation practice. Increase your meditation time by 5 minutes from what you were doing last week—in other words, if you were regularly practicing 15 minutes a day last week, do 20 minutes this week.

Review the practice instructions from last week (page 36). In week 1 you may have explored a number of different focal points for your attention in your sitting meditation. Now choose one of the focal points from week 1 as your anchor and commit to it during week 2. That way you'll have some time to develop a relationship with it.

Suspend any rush to judgment about whether that approach is working. Just settle in and see how it reveals itself to you over the course of the week. You can always change it next week if you wish.

In your seated meditation, dial in the same quality of relaxed, accepting, curious attention that you've been cultivating in your asana practice. Notice the difference in the quality of your sitting meditation after doing a conscious, exploratory asana practice. Remember, it's normal for your attention to drift in and out. When you notice that you've become disconnected from your felt sense of your anchor in your body, don't beat yourself up. Just note that you've been gone—and now you are back. How does your body feel now? Has your thought storm left a trail of physical sensation in its wake? Are you willing to reconnect with the river of your embodied life?

In Your Daily Life This Week

A mindful asana practice is great training for daily life, where much of the time you're not just sitting still receiving experiences but are actively engaged in moving through and manipulating your physical environment. As you're going about your day, play with shifting the lens of your awareness as you walk to and from your car or the bus, shop for groceries, or fold laundry. See if you can keep part of your attention in your body as you engage in conversations or even—ultra-advanced practice—as you work at the computer. Explore your movements through your different activities as an extended vinyasa, a long-form meditation in movement.

RESOURCES

The extraordinary yoga teacher Angela Farmer, with whom I first studied in the early 1990s, has shaped my exploratory, sensate approach to asana practice. Check out her videos and retreats (with her partner, Victor van Kooten) at www.angela-victor.com. For more about the practice of yin yoga and a fusion of Buddha dharma and yoga, go to Sarah Powers's book *Insight Yoga*, her DVDs, and her classes and retreats at www.sarahpowers.com.

Getting to Know Your Breath

A FEW YEARS AGO, five days into a ten-day retreat, a yoga teacher came to me for some help with her meditation practice. She was a petite woman in her midthirties with an athletic asana practice—all week I'd been noticing her calendar-ready poses in our daily yoga sessions as she pressed each pose to its farthest physical limits. Now she perched on the edge of the chair across from me, her hair pulled off her face in a headband, her body poised in perfect yoga-girl posture, with the shoulders flung back and the heart flung forward.

"The teachers keep telling us not to control our breathing—just to be with the breath as it naturally is," she said, visibly agitated. "But I don't have any idea how to do that! What do they mean, 'our natural breath'? How am I *supposed to be breathing?*"

She's not the only one with this question. As yoga practitioners, many of us have been instructed over and over for years on the "right" way to breathe. We've been trained to do a long, slow, controlled breath throughout our asana practice, often involving the technique known as *ujjayi* (literally, the "victorious breath"), in which the back of the throat is constricted slightly to create a soft hiss, like the sound a seashell makes when you hold it up to your ear. We've learned pranayama techniques for altering the length of our breath, the area of the body we're breathing into (belly, chest, side ribs, kidneys), or which nostril we're predominantly breathing through. We've learned to calibrate the ratios of our inhalations and exhalations in formulas that can get so complicated that you wish you had paid more attention in algebra class.

But to just sit still and let the breath breathe itself for hour after hour, giving it our full attention without any intervention whatsoever? That may be terrifying.

At the other end of the spectrum, many Buddhist meditation practitioners have been adamantly informed that they must never manipulate the breath through any kind of conscious breath training lest the fragile edifice of their mindfulness come tumbling down around their ears. When I first started teaching yoga on meditation retreats more than a decade ago, I was warned not to teach any pranayama—the yogic art of breath cultivation—because it would contradict the instructions to observe the breath without interfering with it. If you did pranayama in the meditation hall, it was shocking, as if you had stood up and begun to do a striptease at the back of the room.

Locked into this "don't manipulate the breath" position, mindfulness meditators sometimes persist hour after hour, day after day, year after year, trying to "watch" a breath that is distorted through a lifetime of unconscious patterning—and whose distortions are constantly broadcasting emergency signals to their central nervous system, provoking a dust storm of anxious thinking as their brain tries to plan for the unidentified disaster.

So which approach is right? Do we develop our capacity to be with the breath as it is? Or do we deliberately cultivate ways of working with it?

In my experience, both approaches are what the Buddha called *upaya,* or skillful means—and they can work together to deepen our capacity for awareness, peace, and joy in our meditation and our life. Both, however, have pitfalls that we need to look out for.

In this program we'll embrace a meditative approach to being with the breath that incorporates three dimensions of practice: (1) getting to know the breath, (2) freeing the breath, and (3) enhancing the breath to support emotional balance, well-being, and meditative depth. This week we're going to focus on exploring aspects one and two: getting to know the breath and freeing the breath. Next week we'll continue to free our breath while beginning to practice breath-enhancement techniques.

However, it's important to understand that these are not linear, sequential steps but an ever-changing dance. At different moments you'll emphasize one aspect or another, but they're all part of the same fluid practice—and like holograms, each one contains all the others.

FINDING YOUR NATURAL BREATH

The yogic breathing practices known as pranayama can be a powerful way to balance and settle the energy body and the nervous system in preparation for meditation, creating the conditions in which relaxed attention can flourish. If you're anxious, pranayama can settle you down; if you're sluggish, it can wake you up; if your mind is scattered, it can settle the dust storm of your thoughts.

But if all you know how to do is manipulate your breath, you may be missing important information that your natural, unimpeded breath has to give you. You may be layering on control over a breath that's already distorted or gripped. And in doing so, you block it from unwinding and unleashing the vast potential energy it can offer to your life and practice.

Often when yoga practitioners sit down to meditate, they immediately start doing ujjayi breathing without even realizing it—much to the dismay of the meditators on nearby cushions, who may feel as if they're sitting next to a malfunctioning furnace. Many yoga practitioners are so accustomed to this habitual constriction of the breath that they feel unmoored without it. Addicted to the bliss buzz that can come with a forceful manipulation of the breath, they quickly get bored with—or don't even register—the more subtle sensations that accompany everyday breathing. And when they finally begin to let their breath control go, they are sometimes overwhelmed by the emotions that begin to boil up—which they may have been holding at bay by coercing the breath, that most intimate consort of the unconscious, to obey the stern decrees of the conscious mind.

So before you begin any sort of pranayama practice, it's crucial to cultivate your ability to know the breath without controlling it. You want to enter into a delicate relationship with your breath—which is linked to the deepest layers of your body and psyche—so it can reveal itself without fear of being judged or coerced.

In mindfulness meditation practice, we don't boss our breath around. We don't demand that it be long, deep, slow, or smooth. We don't make it get dressed up in its fanciest clothes and parade down a fashion runway. We get genuinely interested in the way it's showing up right now.

If you can learn to be with a single breath just as it is, without trying to change it, then perhaps you can gradually learn to be with your heart just as it is, or your child or your partner or your best friend.

In his teachings on the Four Foundations of Mindfulness, the Buddha compares the precision with which a practitioner pays attention to his or her breath to a craftsman turning wood on a lathe: "Just as a skilled turner knows when he makes a long turn, 'I am making a long turn,' and knows when he makes a short turn, 'I am making a short turn,' so a practitioner, when he breathes in a long breath, knows, 'I am breathing in a long breath,' and when he breathes in a short breath, knows, 'I am breathing in a short breath'; when she breathes out a long breath, knows, 'I am breathing out a long breath,' and when she breathes out a short breath, knows, 'I am breathing out a short breath.'" Notice that the Buddha does not say that one kind of breath is better than another. What matters here is the care with which the practitioner attends.

When you first start paying attention to your breath this way, your breath might get shy and self-conscious, especially if you've been told to "just let the breath be natural." It's just like when someone whips out a camera, points it straight at you, and says, "Don't pose, just be yourself," and your face immediately freezes into a fake grin or a tense mask of nonchalance. That's okay. Let the breath be awkward. After a while it will forget you are there, the way the contestants on a reality TV show forget they are on the air. It will stop putting on special outfits and makeup and get back to wandering around in its pajamas with its hair uncombed.

It will relax—at least in part—because you have cultivated the art of being friends with it in an undemanding way.

Freeing the Breath

At the same time, it's important to recognize that the breath that you meet when you first sit down to befriend it has already been conditioned in a thousand ways. The breath "just as it is" is shaped by countless factors, from immediate circumstances (you just sprinted up the stairs to catch a ringing phone) to events buried deep in your past (you were left alone to cry yourself to sleep in your crib). For years you may have sucked in your belly to look good in your skinny jeans. Sorrow may have clamped down on your throat or fear on your pelvic floor. Your breath can be frozen from a day in commuter traffic, an angry committee meeting, a belt that's too tight. Or it may hold more chronic contractions from years of abuse, swallowed secrets, and choked-down terrors—patterns that may have been passed down for generations.

This shallow, contorted breath may, without your even being aware of it, be sending constant red alerts to your reptilian brain: *Be afraid! Be very afraid!* This creates even more agitation and an accompanying cascade of opinions, plans, and stories as your mind tries to figure out how to keep you safe.

Ironically, for many of us the very attempt to "concentrate" and control our mind through meditation—and the attendant self-judgment when instead our mind just marches ahead with its own agenda—creates tension in the body and the breath, bringing up more anxiety and rigidity and a corresponding firestorm of thoughts. In an effort to achieve a chimerical ideal of stillness, we don't just perpetuate our usual holding patterns—we add a whole new layer of "meditator freeze" as we attempt to hold our bodies in the "still" position that we think of as appropriate for meditation. Then we struggle to "watch the breath" from the vantage point of our head, cut off from a felt sense of its oceanic tides.

Sometimes, when the breath is constricted in this way, just being with it as it is will allow it to gently unwind in its own time. But sometimes it needs more help than that. If we don't intervene to break the cycle of self-perpetuating tension, we can sit miserably for meditation session after session, never experiencing deep ease.

So it's skillful to work consciously to release the breath as part of your meditation practice—just as skillful as it might be to turn off a radio in the next room or close a window that's blasting icy air. Here's where the tools of yoga asana and pranayama can be invaluable.

It's important to undertake this breath cultivation in a sensitive, intimate, and deeply respectful way. If you leap directly into complex pranayama techniques or even simple instructions such as "take a deep breath," you may layer these patterns on top of an already constricted breath and thereby pave over—without dealing with it—the underlying physical and emotional gripping.

Instead, what you want to do is support yourself in finding your true, free breath—the breath that blows naturally through the forest of your muscles and bones, rustling the leaves. This is not so much a *doing* as an *undoing*. Through gentle exploration, you encourage your unique patterns of constriction to emerge—and then help them unwind.

As you do that, you may discover a whole different way of meditating with your breath. You open into a felt sense of the pulsation of breath throughout your whole body instead of grimly observing it from the outside as it rattles around the prison of your rib cage. You relax into its nourishing, life-giving support. You may begin to sense it as a field of energy that radiates beyond the confines of the physical body, into which you can surrender. And as the breath begins to release, it makes available a cache of vitality that can invigorate not just your practice but your life.

Why Does Breathing Matter?

As meditation teachers are fond of pointing out, the breath is always here and it's always now. Focusing on *this* breath—the felt sensation of it, not the idea of it—can be a present-moment magnet for the iron filings of your scattered attention.

But the reasons to tend to the breath run deeper than that. The breath is the one function of the body that's both voluntary and involuntary, with deep links to both of those branches of the central nervous system.

You can go about your day and the breath will keep on breathing itself, just as your heart keeps beating, your neurons keep firing, your lymph keeps circulating, and your stomach keeps pouring out digestive acids.

And yet you can easily affect this involuntary function—holding the breath, shortening or lengthening it, speeding it up or slowing it down—and by doing so affect other functions normally thought of as involuntary, like heart rate, skin tension, body temperature, and muscle tone. In this way the breath is a bridge between the conscious and the unconscious aspects of our being.

In the yogic view the breath is just one tangible manifestation of the prana, the life force energy that pours through the whole body. So although the term *pranayama* is often thought of as breath practice, it's more accurately considered energy practice. The yogic word for breath—*prana* in Sanskrit, *pana* in Pali—embraces both the physical and the energetic aspects of this pulsation of energy that is with us from the time we are born until the time we die.

Because the layers of our being are interpenetrating fields, when we cultivate balance, steadiness, and ease in the breath, we bring those qualities to the body, mind, and heart as well. Breath is inextricably linked with our physical activities—notice how it changes when you run up the stairs or fall asleep. But it's also linked with our emotions, our dreams, our deepest desires. It's the courier for our fears and passions—we gasp in terror, moan as we make love.

How we are with our breath can reveal how we are with other aspects of our life as well. Do we tend to dominate and control it? Do we space out? By consciously working with our breath, we create an inner environment that is conducive to calming and focusing the heart and mind. And from the perspective of that clear, balanced mind and heart, we can see more clearly into the dharma—the truth of how things are.

THE ANATOMY OF BREATHING

On the physical level, the breath is initiated primarily by the movements of the diaphragm, the lopsided dome of muscle that separates the chest cavity from the abdomen. Directly above the diaphragm sit the heart and lungs. Below the diaphragm are the abdominal organs, including the liver, spleen, stomach, intestines, bladder, and uterus.

When the diaphragm contracts, its dome flattens, creating a vacuum in the lungs that draws the air in. When the diaphragm releases, it rises back up, and the air flows out of the lungs again.

As the diaphragm flattens, it presses down on the abdominal cavity, shifting the abdominal organs. When the abdominal muscles are

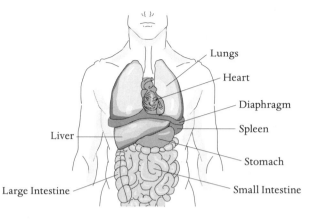

relaxed, the displacement of the organs causes the belly to rise, making more room for the diaphragm to release. When the belly is contracted, the diaphragm can't move as freely, the breath is constricted, and the breathing action is taken over by the smaller—and much less efficient—secondary respiratory muscles of the upper chest, which are primarily designed to kick in in emergency situations.

That's why "breathing into the belly" is often used as a tool for triggering the relaxation response. This full, relaxed breath is more efficient at oxygenating the body—and just as important, it sends a signal to the central nervous system that all is well.

But it's not just the belly that moves in response to the breath. In a relaxed body, the billowing movement of the diaphragm sends ripples out through the whole body, like a pebble dropped into a pond. The entire web of the body—laced together by muscles and fascia—pulses in response to every inhalation and exhalation: pelvic floor widening and releasing, sacrum rocking, spine swaying. Even the bones of the skull subtly dance.

We breathe with our whole body, and hence, when we meditate, we meditate with our whole body.

Sadly, however, most of us block this movement through bodies frozen from trauma and habitual numbness. We harden the tissue around the joints, so they can't move in response to the breath.

And if we don't take the time to unwind these interior layers, we can't really meditate in our bodies. We remain on lockdown in our minds, "watching" the breath struggle within its prison walls.

This week's practices are designed to help us tune in to the delicious pulsation of breath throughout our body, as well as to sense and release the places where this pulsation is blocked.

WEEK 3 PRACTICES

For this week's practices, be especially sure that you are wearing loose-fitting clothing. Unfasten belts and unhook bras. Even many yoga clothes are too snug; especially beware of camisoles that constrict the rib cage.

Before doing any of these breath practices, I highly recommend beginning with a 5- to 15-minute version of Exploring the Whole Body (page 44) to ground yourself in the felt sense of your body so you are not observing the breath from the outside but *feeling* it from the inside—a crucial distinction.

Of course, if you don't have the time or inclination to do a body scan first, you can go straight into the breath-exploration practices. This will enable you to see what your breath—and the quality of your attention—is like with no previous relaxation, which is always useful information.

Each day: Be sure to leave at least 15 minutes for your seated meditation. If you've been regularly practicing 15 minutes, increase it to 20 or 25.

Here are some sample sequences:

Days 1–2: Exploring the Whole Body (5–10 minutes) and Getting to Know the Breath (10–15 minutes). Then move into Opening and Closing the Body with the Breath. Explore this theme of opening and closing through a mindful yoga practice for 15 to 40 minutes using the principles of exploration you investigated in week 2. Complete by returning to Getting to Know the Breath and notice what's changed.

Days 3–5: Touch in with the elements of your breath through Getting to Know the Breath (5 minutes), then explore further with Where Does the Breath Move? (10–15 minutes). Then move into a 20- to 40-minute asana practice that specifically targets areas where you've noticed the breath is frozen, using the tips from In Your Asana Practice This Week (page 91). Experiment with both yin and dynamic sequences. Conclude by returning to Where Does the Breath Move? and noticing what has changed.

Days 6–7: After connecting with your breath through your favorite of the sensing methods you've explored, open the stuck areas through your asana practice. Then practice Inviting the Breath to Move More Deeply.

PRACTICE 3.15
Getting to Know the Breath (10–15 minutes)

🔊 For a guided audio version of this practice, go to www .shambhala.com/movingintomeditation.

You deepen your ability to sense the breath by homing in on four specific aspects: location, length, texture, and the spacing between breaths.

Lie on your back with your knees bent and the soles of the feet on the floor about hip width apart. Experiment with the distance between the feet, and between the heels and the buttocks, until you find a position in which the legs rest with minimal effort. Release the full weight of your body. Relax any extra gripping in the jaw, the muscles around the eyes, the root of the tongue. Soften the skin on your face and belly. If you are pulling your spine away from the floor, surrender it to gravity. Close your eyes. (If it helps you relax, place a silk eye pillow over them.) Without attempting to change the breath in any way, tune in to the sensation of the breath as you begin to explore.

Location. When we breathe, the air itself moves in and out of the lungs—but the *movement* of our breathing can ripple through the tissues of the whole body. Where in your body do you sense the movement of the breath most strongly? If you'd like, you can place one hand on your heart and the other on your lower belly, then rest there for 5 to 10 breaths. Which hand is moving more? Then release your hands by your sides with the palms facing up. Can you still sense the movement of breath in heart and belly? Now which one do you feel most clearly?

Now, for 5 to 10 breath cycles, focus primarily on your exhalation. Where do you first sense the movement of your exhalation? Is it in your nostrils? Your rib cage? Your belly? Your pelvic floor? With each new breath, you may sense your exhalation beginning in a different location. What is the lowest place in your body that you can feel your exhalation begin?

Then turn your attention primarily to your inhalation. Where do you first sense the movement of your inhalation? Where does the movement travel?

Think of the breath movement as having a place from which it emanates, like the ripples from a pebble tossed into a pool. Where is the epicenter of your breath right now? Is it the lower belly? Midbelly? Heart area? Upper chest?

Do you feel the breath most strongly in the front of the body? Or in the back of the body, where it rests against the floor? Does your spine move in response to the breath? How about your rib cage? How about your collarbones? How about the soles of your feet?

Spend about 5 minutes sensing into the places you feel the breath the most. Feel them from the inside, as a river of ever-changing sensation, rather than simply visualizing them. Now imagine that instead of the breath moving inside you, you are resting inside the embrace of a breath that is larger than you, the energy breath that expands in all directions beyond the confines of your skin. How does this change the way you sense the location of the breath?

Length. Now begin to pay attention to the length of your breath. Count the length of each exhalation and inhalation: *One-om. Two-om. Three-om. Four-om.* Don't try to lengthen the breath or make it more uniform. Just notice: How long is each exhalation? How long is each inhalation?

Count for at least 20 complete cycles of inhalation and exhalation (or set a timer and count for 4 or 5 minutes). In general, how long are your inhalations? Are they fairly uniform in length, or do they vary a lot? How long are your exhalations? Are they uniform or varied? Which is usually longer, your inhalation or exhalation?

You'll probably find that the very act of paying attention causes your breath length to change. The breath may become longer. Or it may almost disappear. Don't worry about that: just keep paying attention.

Some people find counting intrusive. If that's the case for you, you can still tune in to the length of the breath on a more intuitive level—using your internal clock to sense, for example, whether your inhalations are shorter or longer than your exhalations. But especially in the beginning, counting helps a lot, and it will be a useful tool to get comfortable with as we work more explicitly with cultivating the breath down the road.

Texture. Now pay attention to the texture of the breath. Is it smooth? Jagged? Steady? Bumpy? Is it faster at the beginning of an inhale or exhale than it is at the end? Does it snag or limp? If your breath were a calligrapher's brushstroke, would it be wider at the beginning and then taper off? Or vice versa? Would it be wavy? Or would it be a uniform stroke from beginning to end?

Spacing. Finally, pay attention to the spaces between the breaths—the slight natural pauses at the top of the inhalation and the bottom of the exhalation. How wide are these gaps? Are they the same length after the exhalation and the inhalation? Are they obvious or almost invisible? Do you find yourself grabbing for the next breath before you've finished the one you're on? Or are there long pauses between each one? If the pauses are long, you might try counting how long they last: *One-om. Two-om. . . .*

Notice what happens to the spaces between breaths as you pay attention to them. Notice what happens to your thoughts.

Going further. When you have completed this exercise, if you have time, flow through a simple, mindful 15- to 20-minute asana practice aimed at loosening the restrictions in your breath (see In Your Asana Practice This Week, page 91). Remember to stay connected throughout with your felt sense of your body. Notice the impact of each asana on the movement of the breath. Then return to the breath-sensing practice again. Take a few minutes to touch again each of the aspects of the breath: location, length, texture, and spacing. How have they changed as a result of your practice?

PRACTICE 3.16
Where Does the Breath Move? (15 minutes)

In this practice you will sense even more finely the movement of breath in the body—where it ripples freely and where it's stuck. In the process, you will naturally begin to release some of the unconscious ways you may be constricting it.

In all of these breath-sensing practices, you are exploring a delicate dance between sensing the breath as it is and inviting it to release. You approach the breath with a gracious invitation to be exactly as it is. Then in an undemanding way you discover how you might be unconsciously restricting its free flow. This is qualitatively very different from demanding change. You are not standing over your breath and making it do a hundred push-ups. Instead, you are holding it in your arms—and letting it hold you—as you dance together.

1. Begin by coming into Child's Pose, kneeling on the floor with your belly resting on your thighs and the knees slightly apart. Relax into your breath. Sense the movement of your belly on your thighs as you breathe. Can you feel the belly expanding on each inhalation? Can you feel the back of the body broadening across the sacrum?

   Now sense the movement of the pelvic floor. In a relaxed body, each inhalation will expand into the perineal area, the soft triangle between the sitting bones, just between the anus and the genitals. This "pelvic diaphragm" mirrors the movement of the respiratory diaphragm. (See the Anatomy of Breathing section on page 79 for a description of how and why this movement happens, and check out the anatomical drawing on page 80.) Can you sense the pelvic floor softening and widening with every inhalation and drawing in with every exhalation? Don't forcibly create this movement. Instead, make room for an inner release that allows this natural movement to happen. Don't worry if you don't feel anything at first. With practice, the release will happen more and more easily. Your intention is to explore what's there rather than create anything special. In this and all of the breath-exploration postures that follow, continue to ask yourself: What would I need to let go of in order to allow the breath to move freely in this area?

2. Now turn onto your back as you were in Getting to Know the Breath (page 82). Continue to sense the movement of the breath in the belly, lower back, and pelvic floor, just as you did in Child's Pose. Sense into the contact of the sacrum with the floor. In a relaxed body, every inhalation will tilt the sacrum so it slopes toward the tailbone. Every exhalation will release it the other way. This rocking is a very subtle movement but a constant one, providing a gentle pulsation that helps circulate the cerebrospinal fluid that bathes and nourishes the brain and the nervous system. It is easily blocked by gripping in the belly, lower back, and pelvis. What needs to release inside you so that you can feel this subtle rocking?

If you place your hands lightly on your pubic bone, you may feel a matching rocking taking place there. Or place them lightly on your outer hips and upper thighs and feel how the breath subtly widens the hips away from each other on every inhalation.

Take your time with this exploration. Be patient and wait for the undoing to occur—don't try to do the undoing. If you're having trouble sensing the rocking of the sacrum, it can sometimes help to create this movement, as we often do in asana practice—deliberately arching the lower back slightly as you inhale and pressing it against the floor as you exhale. This intentional movement may help break up the muscular gripping. But remember: This deliberate action—which comes from muscular activity in the local area of the lower back and sacrum—is not the same as the spontaneous rocking of a relaxed body. What you are looking for is the natural rocking of this area in response to the movement of the diaphragm, which can happen only if the muscles in the lower back and pelvis are relaxed rather than active. So after you've consciously rocked for a few breaths, let that deliberate movement go and return to waiting for the responsive moment of the sacrum that happens with no muscular effort on your part.

3. Now wrap your arms around yourself and place your right palm on the outside of your left shoulder just at the head of the arm bone, and vice versa. Continue to relax and breathe. Can

you sense the shoulders broadening with every inhalation and drawing together on every exhalation? Can you feel the upper back widening between the shoulder blades? (Note: Allowing this natural movement in the upper back to occur as you breathe may spare you much suffering when you sit for long periods in meditation.)

4. Now cradle your skull in your palms. Rest your palms firmly on the bones of the cranium. The seemingly solid skull is in fact composed of multiple bones stitched together by rigid articulations called sutures. Can you feel—or even imagine— the subtle movement of the cranial bones pulsing with the breath? Or are you gripping your skull in an iron band as you try to control the world with your thinking?

   Notice what happens to your sense of the breath in the skull if you deliberately soften the sense organs—the eyes, the inner ears, the root of your tongue, the mouth and jaw (see Feel Your Sense Gateways, page 43). Again, stay here awhile— at least 3 to 5 minutes—and wait. Undo rather than do. Receive rather than chase after sensation.

PRACTICE 3.17
Opening and Closing the Body with the Breath (5–10 minutes)

In this series of practices we'll explore synchronizing some easy opening and closing gestures of the body with the movement of the breath. Pay careful attention to how these movements affect the breath and how the breath affects the movement.

Hands. Sit or lie in a relaxed position with the palms facing up and the backs of the hands supported on the floor or your thighs. As you exhale, slowly and steadily curl the fingers toward the palms into a firm fist. As you inhale, unfurl the fingers until the palm is blossomed wide open. Let the movement last the full length of your breath and pause during the natural space at the top and bottom of the breath. As you did in the practices in week 1, stay connected to the felt sense of the hands moving. Repeat for 15 to 20 breath cycles, then pause. How has this simple gesture affected the quality of your breath—its speed, its texture, its location within your body?

Arms. Lie on your back with your knees bent and the soles of your feet flat on the floor, with your arms resting beside you with the palms facing down. Sweep the arms in front of you and overhead on the inhalation, and release them down on the exhalation. Again, let this movement be steady and smooth. Match the movements to the breath. Let the breath envelop each movement, beginning your inhalations and exhalations slightly before the body begins to move and continuing them until slightly after it rests in stillness again. Count: How long are your inhales while lifting? How long are your exhales while lowering? Use the movement as a tool to smooth out the texture of the breath so that the arms and breath move at a consistent speed, not rushing or lagging at different parts of the arc. This can also be done in a sitting position.

Bridge Pose. Now add movement of the pelvis so that as you inhale and sweep the arms overhead, the pelvis floats up to the sky in a synchronized movement. As you exhale, the arms and pelvis lower back down. Keep the breath smooth and steady and the movements slow. Envelop the movement with the breath. Imagine that your breath energy expands beyond the confines of your physical body, radiating out in all directions with every inhalation and gathering back to the core of your body with every exhalation.

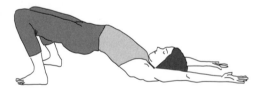

These deceptively simple opening and closing movements ripple through any yoga asana practice. You can practice them in simple gestures such as Cat-Cow or while flowing back and forth between Downward Dog and Upward Dog. Or you can practice them in more dynamic sequences such as Half Sun Salutations or full Sun Salutations. You can explore them in the midst of a strong vinyasa practice as you open and close along with the breath while moving in and out of increasingly demanding postures.

But don't confuse dramatic movements with advanced practice. We are cultivating the ability to notice subtle inner grippings and the unwinding of the breath from the inside out. In more physically demanding postures, you may be so distracted by the muscular exertion—and the sheer fun of the athleticism—that you don't notice where you are holding. So keep it externally simple for now so you can go deeper into the inner journey.

Try this: After exploring opening and closing with the breath, go back to the basic breath-sensing practice (Getting to Know the Breath, page 82). Notice how these movements have affected the length, location, and texture of your breath and the pauses between breaths.

PRACTICE 3.18
Inviting the Breath to Move More Deeply (10–15 minutes)

🔊 For a guided audio version of this practice, go to www
.shambhala.com/movingintomeditation.

We continue our exploration of where the breath moves in the body by consciously inviting the breath to move more freely in various areas. Remember: In doing so you are not dominating the breath. Rather, you are undoing patterns of restriction that block the natural capacity of the breath to flow. As you explore each area, ask yourself: What could I let go of to allow the breath to move here more freely? *This practice will deepen every time you return to it as more and more layers of the body release.*

---

1. Begin by lying on your back with the knees bent, as you did in practice 3.15: Getting to Know the Breath. Take a few minutes to check in with the breath's location, length, texture, and spacing.

   Now place your hands on your lower belly, between the pubic bone and the navel—fingers fanned wide and pointing toward each other. Sense the belly moving under your hands. How big is the movement? Do you feel it more on one side of the belly than the other? Can you feel it in the back body, opposite your hands?

Ask the breath to move more fully into this region. Sense its movement radiating from the lower belly, midway between the pubic bone and the navel, expanding out as a globe of energy and sensation. Imagine that you are drawing the breath directly in and out of the belly. Don't force the movement—instead, melt any obstacle to its happening. What does it feel like to let your breath inhabit this part of your body?

Remember, you are not just expanding the front of the belly. The lower back, kidney area, and sides of the body are also softening to receive the flow of breath. The pelvic floor is widening. With every breath, release a little more to allow the breath to widen and expand out and down. (I picture this as a pear-shaped breath.)

You are not straining to push the breath down into your belly. Rather, you are asking your belly to let go from deep inside. Physiologically, this practice invites the diaphragm to move freely down into the abdominal region while softening the abdominal muscles to allow the organs to move in response to the diaphragmatic action. It encourages the very lowest lobes of the lungs to expand.

From an energetic point of view, breathing into the lower body charges up the hara, the power center of the belly. In yogic anatomy, when you breathe into your pelvic floor, you facilitate the flow of energy through the root chakra, the *muladhara,* which helps anchor and ground your meditations.

2. Now shift the hands upward so they cup the lower floating ribs, with the fingers pointing in toward the bottom tip of the sternum and the thumbs wrapping round toward the kidneys. Your hands are now tracing the edges of the diaphragm, where it attaches to the rib cage and the spine. Invite the breath to open into this area. As you inhale, encourage the breath to open outward, expanding the whole circle of the lower rib cage and widening the diaphragm. Allow the breath to lengthen with every inhalation as you expand the rim of the diaphragm in all directions.

Do the ribs expand evenly and smoothly on both sides? Do

the front and back of the rib cage open equally? Or is the movement uneven? Most people are surprised to discover how the opening lurches from side to side. As you encourage the breath to deepen with each inhalation, intend the expansion of the rib cage—and the widening of the diaphragm—to be as even as possible.

3. Finally, place your hands just under the collarbones, fingers pointing in and thumbs hooking into the armpits to sense the movement of the very top ribs. Encourage your breath to move into this area—expanding into the upper chest. As you did with the lower rib cage, notice whether the very upper rib cage is expanding evenly on both sides and gently encourage it to do so if (as is likely) it isn't. Don't forget to breathe into the back body as well as the front. Can you sense your shoulder girdle slightly expanding with every inhalation? Can you sense the space between the shoulder blades widening?

Stay at each area for at least 3 to 5 minutes. In each area, invite the breath to move as fully as possible, radiating from deep in the body out through the skin and beyond. Ask yourself: How does it feel to breathe from—and into—this part of my body? Is it familiar or unfamiliar? Is there an emotional quality associated with the sensation of the breath in each area?

When you have completed the sequence, take a few long, full breaths in which you consciously expand into each area of the body in turn within each breath—expanding first the lower belly, then the lower rib cage, then the upper chest. Empty completely after each exhalation.

Then rest in the natural breath, receiving it as it ebbs and flows. And again notice: What is its location, length, texture, spacing?

In Your Asana Practice This Week

Yoga poses are tailored to loosen the physical, energetic, and emotional constrictions that can block the free flow of breath. But if your asana practice is mechanical or straining, you won't get the full benefit of these openings. It's possible to perform advanced asanas and still harden the body against the natural pulse of the breath.

So in your asana practice this week, sense into the places where tension lurks: Behind the eyes? In the death grip of the jaws? In a hardened belly, a contracted sphincter?

Energy flows best through a relaxed body. So even when the muscles are working dynamically, keep them pliant. Avoid locking the joints.

Consciously open the parts of the body where you find it more difficult to breathe. Don't come into this with a fix-it attitude. Rather, you're entering into a conversation: Where is the breath asking to move more fully?

If the breath feels stuck in the side ribs, for example, you might explore side bends and twists. If it's stuck in the upper chest, try back bends such as Camel, Wheel, or Bow. If you're having a hard time breathing into your back body, do some long-held yin forward bends such as Seated Forward Bend or Child's Pose. Hip openers such as Baddha Konasana and Pigeon can help move the breath into the pelvic floor. The pelvic floor is also related to the jaw—so release your jaw and the root of your tongue and see if that affects how you sense the breath in the pelvis.

You are deepening your conversation with your body to include not just its more obvious physical movements but also the subtle murmurs of your breath and energy body. So don't smash your body open like a walnut in a nutcracker. Let it melt slowly like ice on a windowpane dissolving in the warm sun of your attention.

In Your Seated Meditation Practice This Week

Be sure to allow at least 20 minutes each day this week for seated meditation. (And if you've regularly been practicing 20 minutes or more, add 5 minutes.) When you have finished a session of breath practices, come to your seated position. Sense the breath moving in the specific areas you have been exploring: the pelvic floor, the lower belly, the back body, the skull. Notice its length, spacing, and texture. Are you clenching the body to stay upright? Instead, relax as much as possible.

Investigate where the breath is and isn't moving. Can you still feel the subtle rocking of the sacrum? How about the broadening of the upper back and shoulders? Does the spine sway with the inhales and exhales?

Now let your attention naturally magnetize around one aspect or location of the breath: the belly moving in and out as the diaphragm billows up and down, the pelvic floor softly opening and closing in synchrony with the diaphragmatic movements, the prickle of the breath in the nostrils, the natural pauses at the top of the inhale and the bottom of the exhale, the whole body being breathed.

Whatever you choose, rest with it as your anchor—not as a concept but as a living caress. When your mind drifts off, invite the feeling of breath to rise up and fill your attention—sensual, alive, and ever-changing. Remember that meditative presence is not something you need to strain to create. It's always right there waiting for you, under the frantic busyness of all of your scheming and projects.

For just this short time, give yourself a respite from the thunder of your plans, the squeaks and scurries of your worries. Be grounded and soothed by each breath out, nourished and enlivened by each breath in.

In Your Daily Life This Week

As you move through your daily activities, pause periodically to notice your breath. Set a timer on your computer or phone to chime every couple of hours. When it does, pause and feel into the four aspects of your breath at that moment—its location, length, texture, and spacing. Is there anywhere you are holding your body tight against the natural flow of your breath? Is there somewhere you can let go—in your body or in your mind—that would free your breath?

RESOURCES

Donna Farhi's *The Breathing Book* is the bible for anyone wanting to get to know the freedom of the unconditioned breath. Many of the breath practices in this chapter are variations of techniques I originally learned from her masterful teaching. Thich Nhat Hanh's translation of the Anapanasati Sutra, *Breathe, You Are Alive: The Sutra on the Full Awareness of Breathing,* breathes fresh life into this classic Buddhist manual on breathing and practice.

WEEK 4

Cultivating Your Breath

WHEN MY SON, Skye, was nine years old, he began getting head-aches—not the ordinary headaches I was familiar with but roll-around-on-the-floor, clutch-your-head-screaming monsters.

Once they got a grip on him, nothing in my medicine cabinet—from homeopathic tinctures to good old Advil—could cut them short. (Nor, I found, did it help very much if I started to cry as well.) Acu-puncture, cranial osteopathy, vision therapy, foot and head massages in a darkened room—nothing worked. Of course, the more he sobbed and struggled, the worse the pain got. "On a scale of one to ten, how bad is it?" I asked him once. "It's an eleven," he moaned.

After the scale-eleven headache, I made an appointment with the Pediatric Headache Clinic in San Francisco. A neurologist interviewed Skye in detail (an experience that left him, predictably, with a throb-bing head). I expected the doctor to send us straight for an MRI. But to my surprise, instead he diagnosed migraines and prescribed bio-feedback.

At Skye's first session, the biofeedback trainer wrapped Skye's abdomen with a belt embedded with electronic sensors hooked up to a computer monitor. She showed him how to make the belt rise and fall by breathing into his belly—thereby drawing beautiful colored waves on the computer screen. Then she taught him how to increase the height and depth of the waves, as well as the distance between them, by deepening and slowing his breath.

Over the next few sessions, Skye learned how to lower his blood pressure, raise and lower his body temperature, relax his skin and muscle tension, slow down his heart rate, and alter his brain wave patterns—all through consciously regulating his breathing patterns. After five or six sessions of biofeedback, the frequency and intensity of his headaches had dramatically lessened. He learned to catch the early warning signs and intervene before they ballooned. Even better, he learned to notice the signs of stress in his breath and body and alter his behavior.

Now when he feels a migraine coming on, he takes a break and lies down in a dark, quiet room to bring his nervous system back into balance, using the deep breathing and relaxation skills that have become second nature to him. He goes months at a stretch between headaches. And it's been years since he's had a real screamer of a migraine.

Skye's story is just one example of the power of conscious breathing. Modern science has corroborated what the yogis have known for centuries—that our breath both reflects and shapes the state of our body and mind.

Yogis have observed that when a practitioner is deep in meditation, the breath often becomes more and more slow and subtle, just as the meditator's capacity to be absorbed in it naturally deepens. As the mind grows still, sometimes the breath suspends for long periods of time—without any effort. So over the centuries, yogis began to inquire: What happens to my meditations if I consciously intervene to slow down the breath? How about if I speed it up and make it more forceful? What if I suspend it entirely?

As it turns out, yogis discovered, it's possible to skillfully support the deepening of meditative presence by consciously intervening in our breathing patterns. Last week we worked with getting to know our breath and freeing our breath as two parts of a three-pronged approach to contemplative breath work. You experienced how noticing ways that you are unconsciously restricting the breath can—just by itself—start to break up those patterns.

This week we'll build on those explorations through conscious breathing patterns that can further liberate the breath from its habitual contractions—while adding a third element, of cultivating the breath, to deliberately increase qualities of energy and relaxation that can support our meditative journey.

In particular we'll explore the way that consciously altering the four qualities of the breath we explored in the last chapter—location, length, texture, and spacing—can deepen our meditation. You'll have the opportunity to sense directly, from the inside out, how this breath cultivation affects your access to mindful presence and inner investigation.

THE ART OF PRANAYAMA

In most contemporary Western yoga classes, pranayama—the art of working with the breath to affect consciousness—generally takes a backseat to the showier asana practices. Even teachers who honor the power of pranayama are typically forced by the confines of the standard ninety-minute yoga class, and the understandable demands of their students for a fitness workout, to limit pranayama to a few minutes at the end of the session lest they lose the majority of their clientele (and subsequently their studio jobs as well).

But if you're interested in yoga as a meditative discipline, it's essential to put pranayama at the core of your practice—increasing not just the frequency with which you practice it but the percentage of your total practice time.

You can use the breath simply as an anchor for your meditation, strengthening your capacity for sustained presence by returning your attention to it again and again. But you'll also discover that *how* you breathe can directly affect the quality of your attention as well as your ability to move into deepened states of absorption.

On the most basic level, scientific research has proven that slowing and deepening the breath activate the parasympathetic nervous system, triggering a set of physiological and mental phenomena that are collectively known as the relaxation response. Heart rate drops. Blood pressure lowers. Muscle and skin tension decrease. Receptors in the nerves and organs coordinate the elements of the body that manage the autonomic nervous system—heart, lungs, limbic system, and cortex—to put your nervous system into a state of balance. In his teachings on the Four Foundations of Mindfulness, the Buddha alludes to this power: "Breathing in, I calm the activities of my body. Breathing out, I calm the activities of my body."

A decrease in breathing frequency increases the synchronization of brain waves as well as boosting the delta waves that are dominant during deep sleep and meditation. An even, deep breath is associated with a mind that is calm, steady, and able to concentrate. One explanation for this shift appears to be the fact that slow breathing dramatically elevates carbon dioxide levels in the blood, effectively drugging the brain into serenity. Other studies indicate that receptors in the respiratory tissues themselves signal the central nervous system to shift gears as the breathing slows down.

On the opposite end of the spectrum, rapid breathing activates the sympathetic nervous system, preparing the body for "fight or flight." The heart speeds up, the muscles tense, and the nervous system moves toward high alert, with all senses scanning the territory for incoming threats. (This tendency can be harnessed skillfully through forceful yet relaxed breathing practices such as *kapalabhati,* the yogic "breath of fire," which studies have shown to brighten mental acuity and visual perception.)

Over time, in meditation the breath tends to settle and slow on its own as the body and nervous system unwind, naturally facilitating this shift from sympathetic to parasympathetic. And as the breath slows, it signals the body that it's safe to relax even more, creating a positive feedback loop.

Deliberately supporting this natural unwinding—through simple yogic pranayama practices—can bring you into a more sensitive and informed relationship with your breath. At the same time, it opens new territory for the breath to move into, leading to the possibility of even deeper releases.

From a traditional yogic perspective, the practices in this chapter derive much of their power from the way they channel the subtle energies in the body. Over centuries of experimentation, yogis concluded that inhalations are characterized by what they call *brahmana* energy— heating, expansive, and energizing. Modern scientific research shows that every time you inhale, your heart rate slightly increases. Every time you exhale, your heart rate slightly decreases.

So if you're feeling sluggish in your meditation, it's skillful to employ pranayama techniques that emphasize the inhalations and the pauses after the inhalations.

The exhalation manifests what's called *langhana* energy: calming and grounding. So if you're feeling anxious or overstimulated, do practices that emphasize the exhalation and the pauses after the exhalation. Longer exhales mean a longer period of time when your heart rate is dropping.

And highlighting the pauses themselves—through the practice known as *kumbhaka,* or breath suspension—also has potent effects on the body and mind. Studies have shown that breath retention after inhalation, for example, increases the dominance of the blissful theta brain waves. In my experience, lengthening the pause after exhalation can be even more powerful, with attendant feelings of calm and inner release.

But don't just take the yogis'—or the scientists'—word for it. Check out these practices in the laboratory of your own body and mind. Once you know them from the inside out, you'll be able to use them intelligently to support your own meditation practice.

Directly engaging with the breath in this way can be an appealing entryway into meditation. For many people it's easier to get—and stay—focused on the breath if they are doing something with it. Once that initial connection deepens into a relationship, you can let go of guiding the breath and let the breath guide you instead—without drifting off and spacing out. You let go of doing but retain the quality of rapt attentiveness.

And consciously working with your breath can be a potent tool when confronting the classic Buddhist hindrances to meditation. Dozing off on your cushion in the grip of a sleepiness attack? Skillful pranayama can brighten your energy. A firestorm of thoughts fanned by winds of anxiety? A different kind of pranayama can put out the flames. (We'll investigate this pattern in greater depth in week 10.)

But it's important to remember that you are not controlling the breath so much as inviting it. Sometimes you lead the breath with your intention, sometimes you follow it wherever it goes—and it's vital to be able to choose when you are leading and when you are following. So after each period of conscious breath work, be sure to return to an uncontrolled breath. Feel from the inside the difference between guiding the breath and just letting it move on its own. See what new freedom your breath has to swirl about inside you as it whispers its way into new territory.

Keep a light hand on the reins. Your breath is not a hired hack pony plodding around the same dusty track. It's a thoroughbred steed—spirited, powerful, and sensitive. Offer it respectful suggestions and sense the signals it gives you in return.

And at the end of a practice, just let the reins go and let it find its own way home.

WEEK 4 PRACTICES

Yogic pranayama is a vast art that you could easily spend years exploring. From the immense array of potential practices, I've picked out a few simple but powerful ones that I have personally found especially helpful in supporting the deepening of meditative practice. The influence of breath practice on meditation does not increase with complexity; from a meditative perspective, you're better off going deeper into a few forms than piling your shopping cart full of breathing tricks.

Don't try to do too many different practices in one session. Just choose one or two to go into deeply and then sit in meditation to soak in the effects. Trying to combine multiple pranayama practices, with a range of energetic effects, in a single session is like trying to spice up a bland soup by adding salt, then curry powder and ginger, then basil and oregano, then soy sauce and wasabi, then a splash of red wine. Best to add one or two spices, taste it, and savor the effects. You can try another combination the next day.

Setup. Try each of the breathing practices in a comfortable reclining position with the spine in its natural curves. The legs can be extended, or the knees can be bent, with the soles of the feet flat on the floor. While pranayama bolsters can be helpful for expanding the diaphragm and rib cage, for our purposes this week it's more useful to have the spine in its natural alignment. Once you've gotten familiar with the practices while reclining, you can try them in a seated position—for most people this is more challenging because of the unconscious muscular constrictions that tend to kick in as soon as we sit upright.

Before you begin. Start each session with the basic reclining practice of Arriving in Your Body (page 38). Take 2 or 3 minutes to feel your way through your body to heighten your sensitivity. Then spend another 2 or 3 minutes assessing the four aspects of your breath that we explored in week 3: location, length, texture, and spacing (Getting to Know the Breath, page 82). This way you'll have a better connection to how your breath is naturally expressing itself in this moment.

Sample practice schedule. The practices are organized according to the way they work with these four aspects of your breath. One way to explore them is to work with a different aspect each day.

Be sure to include at least 20 to 25 minutes of sitting meditation each day. Here's a suggested sequence:

Day 1: Extending the Pause after Exhalation, Extending the Pause after Inhalation, and Extending the Full Pause and the Empty Pause Together.

Day 2: Snake Breath, Lengthening the Exhalation, and Lengthening the Inhalation.

Day 3: Equalizing Inhalations and Exhalations.

Day 4: Continue your work with any two or three of the previous practices and also experiment with Smoothing Out the Breath.

Days 5–7: Choose practices based on your energy. If you are

feeling a little sluggish, choose practices that emphasize the inhalation and the pause after the inhalation. If revved up or anxious, select practices that emphasize the exhalation and the pause after the exhalation.

Experiment with doing your pranayama before your asana practice one day and after your asana practice another day. Notice the difference.

As you'll discover in the following three practices, opening up the pause between breaths has powerful effects on the whole nervous system.

PRACTICE 4.19
Extending the Pause after Exhalation (5–15 minutes)

🔊 For a guided audio version of this practice, go to www.shambhala.com/movingintomeditation.

On days when you are agitated and your mind is busy, this is one of the best ways I know to settle the nervous system and steady the mind.

As you rest in your natural breath, begin to pay particular attention to the slight natural pause after the exhalation. Let yourself fall into it, as if sliding down the long slide of the exhalation and then dropping into the deep pool of the pause. Notice the empty pause before you resurface and inhale again. What happens to the thoughts in that pause? What happens to your sense of self?

Now begin to lightly lengthen that pause—just 2 counts at first: *One-om. Two-om.* You may find, when you do that, that you were not quite done exhaling after all. If that's the case, let a little more breath flow out, then pause again. You might need to repeat that process several times before you have truly exhaled completely. Then let the inhalation flow in on its own without controlling it in any way.

Notice *how* you are pausing. Are you clenching your body to put on the brakes and "hold" the breath out? You may notice some gripping in the throat and the diaphragm, as if you are forcibly holding the breath out—this may manifest not during the pause but in the moment after you begin to inhale, as if you were lurching or gasping your way into the next breath. Instead, just dismantle the action that leads to the inhalation—so that you are *undoing into* the pause rather than *doing* the pause.

In the pause, soften the jaw. The backs of the eyes. The pelvic floor. Where else are you holding tight?

This practice illuminates any tendency to grab for the next breath before you have fully let go of the one before—shining light on the way we continually lean into the next moment. When we allow each exhalation to complete fully, and rest in the pause before breathing in again, we feel ourselves settling back into the present.

You will probably notice that as soon as you deliberately lengthen the pause after the exhalation, the inhalation naturally lengthens on its own. The exhalation, too, may begin to lengthen and smooth out. Do not try to make this happen but do not inhibit it either.

After a few rounds like this, extend the pause still further, by 3 counts. Then 4. Then 5. Then 6. For each increase, practice a few rounds of breath before moving to the next. Notice whether you are subtly rushing your exhalations to get to the pause, which you may perceive as the "point" of the practice, your opportunity to "do something." It's not about pressing ahead to your maximum-length pause, especially since you are doing this with the intention of supporting meditative awakening rather than lung capacity. Rather, it's about creating a meditative rhythm that draws your attention deeper and deeper inward to rest in the silent space between breaths.

Notice how the breath empties into stillness and arises out of stillness, again and again. What happens to the thoughts during this space? What happens to the emotions?

Now let the breathing return to normal. Be sure you take a few minutes to rest with the natural breath so you can really feel the difference between guiding the breath and simply sensing the breath. Continue to attend to the space between the exhalation and inhalation: Is it longer than before? Shorter? The same? What effects do you notice on your energy and mood?

Going further. Once you've gained some familiarity with this practice, begin to notice more subtleties: for instance, the moment when you start to inhale again. Do you grab at the breath greedily to suck it in? Or do you simply allow the inhale to breathe itself?

After you've gotten comfortable with a 6-count hold after exhalation, try extending the suspension beyond that. Rather than counting, just extend the pause but release any effort—just wait for the breath to roll in whenever it's ready, a gentle and inexorable tide.

Notice your quality of being in this empty space of nondoing. If you find yourself gasping at the inhalation, you've forced the hold too long.

After a few minutes of practice, let go of any attempt to guide the breath. Let it return to its natural rhythms. But retain that attitude of waiting for the breath to come to you rather than chasing after it.

PRACTICE 4.20
Extending the Pause after Inhalation (5–10 minutes)

If you're feeling sluggish—especially right before a meditation session—this practice can brighten your attention.

Begin by paying attention to the natural pause after the inhalation— like a wave cresting before tumbling over.

Now expand this pause 1 or 2 counts at a time, just as you did with your pause after exhalation. This is not a tense holding; rather, it's a delicate suspension. In this full pause, imagine the energy of the inhalation, the prana, permeating your entire body. After each hold, let the exhalation flow out.

If you are tensing your jaw or neck in order to "hold" the breath, relax this effort. If you start to feel any dizziness, pressure in the head or eyes, or light-headedness, immediately back off to a shorter count or let the practice go.

When you've extended the inhalation to about 6 counts, take a few minutes to rest in the natural breath and fully absorb the effects of the practice. Notice whether the length of the natural inhalation or exhalation has changed at all. Notice whether the pauses between the breath have expanded.

Going further. Once you've become comfortable with this suspension, explore: What is happening internally at that moment you decide to exhale? Is there any unnecessary pushing or gasping around that moment, any way in which you're forcing your exhalation unnecessarily?

If you're at ease with a 6-count pause, see what happens if you suspend the breath and just wait for the exhalation to release spontaneously.

PRACTICE 4.21
Extending the Full Pause and the Empty Pause Together
(15 minutes)

Once you've explored practices 4.19 and 4.20 and are comfortable with pausing either before or after the inhalation, play with extending both pauses in the same practice. Simultaneously grounding and energizing, this pranayama creates a sense of inner spaciousness by heightening your awareness of the space that surrounds every breath.

Tune in to the four-part rhythm of the breath—the inhalation and the full pause at its top, the exhalation and the empty pause at its bottom. Then begin to lengthen each pause in the same progressive fashion as you did in practices 4.19 and 4.20—adding a count at a time until you've reached 5 or 6 counts. Keep the inhales and exhales smooth (but don't try to control their length for now). If they start to get jagged, back off to a lower count. You're not controlling your breath so much as dancing with it, inviting it to move to a steady pulse of your inner metronome.

You will probably notice that as you work with the pauses, the exhalations and inhalations begin to lengthen and even out on their own. If this happens, allow it—but don't try for it.

Let the even rhythm of the breath soothe you, nourish you, sustain you. Notice how the breath arises out of nothing and dissolves into nothing, again and again.

Going further. As you deepen your work with the pauses between breaths, begin to notice the pauses between thoughts, sensations, and emotions. They, too, arise out of nowhere, dissolve back into nowhere. Pay more attention to the spaces between them than to the thoughts, emotions, and sensations themselves.

You might think that your mind is busy. But as you pay more attention, you begin to see that between thoughts it is not busy at all. Your heart may be filled with sorrow. But what is the state of your heart in that moment when sorrow has passed and no new feeling has yet arisen?

Get very interested in this space.

You may have noticed in the previous practices that when you extended the pause after the exhale, the inhale began to lengthen; when you extended the pause after the inhale, the exhale lengthened. In the following practices, we'll begin to deliberately extend the inhalations and exhalations directly.

PRACTICE 4.22
Snake Breath (5 minutes)

This is a powerful practice for emphasizing and extending the exhalation—a soothing, centering, and grounding practice that's a great way to begin either an asana or a meditation session, especially if you're feeling anxious or agitated. It's much more effective than simply ordering yourself to take a deep breath—although, like all practices that lengthen the exhale, it will immediately have an effect on the depth of your inhalation as well.

In your reclining position, inhale through the nose and then exhale through the mouth with a hissing sound like a snake, letting the breath pass over the tip of the tongue. Hiss your breath all the way out, expelling the last bit of air from the lungs—not by compressing the chest but by drawing in the very lowest part of the belly, just above the pubic bone, as if you were squeezing toothpaste from the bottom of a tube.

When you have completed the exhale, let the inhale naturally flow in.

Repeat for 5 to 10 cycles, emphasizing the drawing in of the lower belly back toward the spine. The hissing naturally slows and regulates the breath and makes its texture audible. Can you keep the sound steady and smooth?

When you have finished, let the breath return to normal. Sense the effect of the practice on the breath, the mind, and the energy body, especially any feeling of warmth or tingling in the lower belly.

PRACTICE 4.23
Inviting the Breath to Lengthen in Movement (5 minutes)

Many people find it easier to lengthen the inhalations and exhalations while engaged in simple movements rather than just focusing on the breath alone. In this practice you'll use repetitive movements of the arms to invite the breath to lengthen. The arm movements naturally create more space in the rib cage for the breath to move into. They also provide a tangible external reference point for the rhythm of the breath.

Begin flat on your back with the knees bent, hip width apart. After checking in with your breath as it is, begin to sweep the arms up overhead and back down as you did in week 3, Opening and Closing the Body with the Breath (page 87).

Sweep the arms in front of you and overhead on the inhalation, and release them down by your side on the exhalation. Match the smooth, steady movements to the breath. Envelop each movement with breath, beginning the inhalations and exhalations slightly before the body begins to move and continuing them until slightly after it rests in stillness again.

Now count: How long are your inhales while lifting? How long are your exhales while lowering? Equalize the length of the inhalations and exhalations at the lower count. If you are naturally inhaling for 4 and exhaling for 6, stabilize them both at 4. Use the movement as a tool to smooth out the texture of the breath—so that arms and breath move at a consistent speed, not rushing or lagging at any part of the arc.

Now lengthen both inhalation and exhalation by 2 counts. If that feels comfortable, after a breath or two elongate them by 2 counts more. Continue this practice until you start to feel any sense of strain or discomfort—then back off to 1 lower count, or 2 if necessary. Breathe this way for a few more cycles, then stop and notice the effect on the breath.

PRACTICE 4.24
Lengthening the Exhalation (5–10 minutes)

Lengthening the exhalations calms the nervous system and can help quiet a busy mind.

In a reclining position, count the length of your natural inhalation and exhalation. Then begin to gradually increase the length of your exhale, 1 or 2 counts at a time.

Imagine regulating the flow of water from a faucet by slightly narrowing the pipe so that the water flows out more slowly. Pay particular attention to the texture of the breath as you extend the exhale. Are you stopping and starting the exhalation like a beginning driver tapping the brake?

Let each inhalation come in naturally, without counting (as counting it will automatically begin to regulate it). Even without counting, you will probably notice that the inhalation gets longer as you slow your exhalation—and that as the inhalation deepens, it naturally becomes easier to draw out the exhalation longer, since you have a greater volume of air to exhale. You may sense, after a few breath cycles, that the air billows back in on the inhalation in a fuller way, expanding the side ribs and upper chest as the diaphragm rebounds downward.

Let the rhythm of the exhalation empty you of the relentless grip of your plans and memories. With each emptying of your lungs, release your body a little more deeply into the earth. Ask yourself with each exhalation: What can I let go of?

Extend the exhalation a little at a time over the course of about 5 minutes. When you've reached your maximum comfortable length, then let the practice go. Notice what happens to the breath. How does it move inside the space you've created? What's the quality of your heart and mind?

PRACTICE 4.25
Lengthening the Inhalation (5–10 minutes)

◀) For a guided audio version of this practice, go to www
.shambhala.com/movingintomeditation.

When instructed to lengthen their inhalation, most people will immediately tense their bodies and start to draw the breath high into the chest—lengthening the breath vertically, as though pouring more water into a thin tube. But what we're interested in here is allowing the breath to deepen by expanding—widening and deepening through the belly, side body, and back as well as filling higher into the chest.

So before you begin to work with lengthening the count of the inhalation, please review the practice you did last week: Inviting the Breath to Move More Deeply (page 89). Once you have reminded yourself of the various ways your breath can expand within your body, you're ready to explore consciously extending the length of your inhalation.

First, in a comfortable reclining position, count the natural length of your inhalations. Then—just as you did with the exhalation in the previous practice—begin to lengthen them, a count or two at a time.

Notice what you reflexively do to make the breath longer. Instead, can you encourage the breath to deepen by *doing less*?

Instead of lengthening the breath by immediately inflating the chest and rib cage, as might be your inclination, begin by letting the breath expand into the belly and lower back. See how many counts you can get to while keeping the breath primarily moving into these areas.

As the breath grows longer, it will naturally expand higher in the body. The epicenter of the breath will shift upward. Notice at what count that happens for you today. Four? Five? Six? Seven? It will change with time. Don't strain. When it feels natural, allow the rib cage to balloon outward as the breath expands into the midbody. Eventually, the breath will expand from the pelvic floor all the way to the tips of the collarbones.

At first you may find that there's a jerky transition as the breath expands from the lower body up and out into the rib cage. Just notice that and relax. With time, as the body softens and releases, that transition will become more and more smooth.

Keep the jaw and eyes soft. Don't control the exhalations. If you notice any strain or light-headedness, let the practice go.

When you have reached your maximum capacity, breathe several rounds at that length. Then return to your natural breath. Observe the effects. Is the inhalation naturally longer now? Do you have a sense of more inner space for the breath to move? Let go of any lingering impulse toward control.

Variation. For some people, it's challenging, and even anxiety provoking, to try to guide the location of the breath at the same time they're focusing on extending its length. They find that their breath feels mechanical and forced. If that's the case for you, let go of that aspect of the exploration. It's meant as a useful support, not another way to try to get things right.

Instead, as you extend the length of your inhalations, just sense the breath expanding and opening in all directions. Instead of picturing the breath filling you from the bottom up, like water pouring into a glass, envision it expanding from the center as if you were blowing up a balloon—radiating beyond the boundaries of the skin in an ever-widening field of energy. Instead of the breath moving inside you, sense yourself resting within the expanding breath.

PRACTICE 4.26
Equalizing Inhalations and Exhalations (15 minutes)

After you have gotten familiar with lengthening the inhalations and exhalations separately, you can move on to lengthening them at the same time.

The object of this practice is not to see how long you can make the breaths. It's to establish an even rhythm of inhale and exhale and then sustain that for several minutes before moving on to a longer rhythm.

Begin, as always, by observing the natural rhythm and duration of your breath at this time. Then pick a comfortable length to work with—for most people, anywhere from 4 to 6 counts is a good length to start at, but yours may be longer, especially if you're a longtime yoga practitioner. Let your breath settle into a steady rhythm around that count. Even if you can comfortably inhale and exhale with a longer count, it's good to begin with a lower count so you can focus on letting the epicenter of the breath be in the belly, or hara. Practice "pear-shaped" breathing: sensing the breath as energy moving in and out of the hara, expanding in all directions beyond the skin. Settle the breath into a steady rhythm around that count for 3 or 4 minutes— long enough that you can relax into it.

Surrender into the rhythm of the breath and find freedom within it. You are deliberately carving out new territory within yourself. Don't view the rhythm as a cage that you are putting your breath inside but, rather, as a drumbeat that the music of your breath can play to.

After 3 or 4 minutes, add a count to both the exhale and the inhale and continue.

Practice this for about 12 to 15 minutes, then release the control of the breath and let it settle into its own natural rhythm. Observe how the breath moves within the new territory that you have carved out. Are you following the breath with the same intimate absorption now that you are no longer trying to do something with it?

Each day that you practice this, try starting with a slightly longer breath. So if the first day you do 5, 6, and 7 counts, the next day try 6, 7, and 8; then 7, 8, and 9. If you start to experience strain at the higher levels of the sequence, then immediately drop back to a lower count. The next day, start your sequence one lower and practice there for a few weeks until you are ready to lengthen.

Note: This is a great practice to do at the start of a meditation period. After doing this practice for 10 to 12 minutes, sit in meditation— absorbed in the sensation of the natural, uncontrolled breath—for at least as long as you practiced the regulated breath. Notice the difference in the quality of your attention when you are directing your breath versus when you are simply allowing it to be. Which is easier for you?

Variation. One of the challenges of counting your breath length is that it's so subjective—your counting speed may vary wildly from breath to breath or even slow down as your breath slows down. For that reason it can be very helpful to use a metronome-like timer that chimes at a regular interval. There is a variety of such timers available, some of them as smartphone apps.

🔊 To download my favorite breath timer—which uses a series of meditation bells designed for this purpose—go to qigong dharma.com/breathintervals. There you will also find instructions for working skillfully with timed breath intervals.

The last aspect of the breath we're going to work with this week is texture—the smoothness of the inhalation and exhalation.

PRACTICE 4.27
Smoothing Out the Breath (5–10 minutes)

When you make the breath audible, it's easier to observe its texture.

The texture of the breath is intimately entwined with its length. So to begin with, come into your rest position on your back and take a few minutes to settle into an even breath rhythm, with inhalations and exhalations approximately the same length (although it's not necessary to count) and a length that you know you can comfortably sustain for 5 or 10 minutes. Now add in the familiar practice of ujjayi—slightly closing the back of the throat so that you hear the oceanic sound of the breath as it moves in and out.

Now begin to focus more precisely on the texture of the breath as it moves in and out, which will be beautifully mirrored in the sound of the breath. Is it steady from beginning to end? Does it jerk and waver?

To heighten your ability to sense the texture of your breath, close the ears with your fingers or with earplugs while you do your ujjayi breathing. Instantly the sound will be amplified to an oceanic rush that seems to be happening not just in your ears but at the very center of your skull. You will hear every jagged edge and bump.

As you become absorbed in this oceanic sound, smooth it out. And sense your mind smoothing out as well.

When you've finished, unplug your ears. Let go of the ujjayi and of any attempt to regulate the breath. As the sound of the breath becomes more subtle, can your attention become more subtle too, to match it?

In Your Asana Practice This Week

In your asana practice this week, continue to explore the power of consciously regulating the texture, length, and spacing of the breath. Notice what happens if you open out the pause between breaths while holding a posture or while flowing through a simple vinyasa sequence.

Establishing a rhythmic count and sustaining it through relatively simple sequences are a powerful way to regulate the nervous system.

In a vinyasa flow, yogis are often instructed to regulate the breath at about a 5-second inhalation and exhalation. However, our subjective sense of how long that is is often distorted, particularly as we begin to heat up the body, move more quickly, and include more physically demanding postures. Often these "advancements" are accompanied by a sped-up or ragged breath. Using a timer can be a powerful, objective tool for regulating the breath at an even pace while you are in motion, increasing your depth of meditative absorption in your vinyasa practice.

In Your Seated Meditation This Week

All of the breathing practices we have covered in this week's practices are easiest to learn lying down. However, once you're familiar with them in a lying-down position, try them in a comfortable seated position.

Notice the difference in your experience when you do these practices sitting up. What is more challenging about it? What is easier? Notice whether the breath feels constricted in different areas from when you were lying down. Notice whether you're gripping in a different way or if overefforting creeps into the breath more strongly.

After each period of breath work—whether reclining or seated—be sure to allow time for a period of seated meditation in which you receive the breath without directing it in any way.

This week, increase your seated meditation time to at least 20 to 25 minutes. What differences do you notice between the felt sense in your body and breath when you are directing the breath and when you are just receiving it? Is it easier for you to pay attention to the breath when you are directing it or when you are just receiving it? Why?

Wherever you sense the breath most strongly, let that be the anchor point for your attention. Rest inside it. Come home to it again and again.

In Your Daily Life This Week

Pay attention to the pauses between breaths as you go through your day—especially the pause after the exhalations. Notice, as your day gets busy, whether you're galloping from one breath to the next without fully exhaling. Take a few minutes to practice lengthening that pause before moving on to your next activity.

Also notice the feeling in your breath when you build in pauses between events, between conversations, between items on your to-do list. Build a little space into your schedule instead of filling every moment with tasks. Notice how that affects your breath as well.

RESOURCES

For a sensitive, thoughtful, and enjoyable exploration of traditional yogic breath practices, turn to Richard Rosen's books *The Yoga of Breath* and *Pranayama beyond the Fundamentals*. I continue to learn something new every time I try one of his practices.

Taking Your Seat

BEFORE YOU BEGIN this chapter, a bit of bad news: if you wait to meditate until you have enough time, you'll probably never do it.

You may imagine that you'll have enough time after you've checked the last item off your to-do list: after you've changed the cat litter and browsed the headlines online and stopped global warming and looked at the profiles of everyone who has winked at you on your dating site, after you've prepared your presentation for tomorrow's meeting and made split pea soup and helped your kids with their math homework (for which you've had to relearn how to multiply fractions, something you had thought you were forever safe from after majoring in art history).

Unfortunately, your list will keep sprouting new Medusa-like heads for every one you cut off. But here's the good news: you can meditate anyway. As one of my Zen teachers, Fu Schroeder, said to me when I was a harried new mother and despaired of finding time to meditate, "How do you have time to do anything else?"

This week we're going to dive more deeply into the art of seated meditation—the classic and powerful meditation form that's been the centerpiece of yogic practice for millennia. The oldest known image of yoga is a five-thousand-year-old clay seal—dug up in the ruins of the ancient Indus Valley city of Harappa—depicting a yogi seated in a cross-legged position. When Patanjali referred to *asana* in his Yoga Sutra, he meant this seated posture, not the pantheon of athletic poses we practice today. The word *asana* actually comes from the Sanskrit verb *as,* "to sit."

Of course, all the explorations of body and breath we have done together in the last four weeks have not just been a preparation for meditation—they are forms of meditation in their own right. And you've been doing a daily sitting practice all along. This week we'll explore refinements in posture and technique that will make it easier for you to sit for longer periods so you can practice a more sustained cultivation of presence and insight that builds upon all the tools of body and breath awareness that you've been developing and deepening over the past month.

For this reason, for the remaining weeks of this program, please make sure that you set aside at least 30 to 45 minutes a day for your seated practice in addition to any asana or pranayama practice you may want to be doing. It's worth *making* the time for, even if you don't already have it. Write it in your calendar. Get up a little earlier, if you have to, or go to bed a little later. And here's some more good news: when you meditate, you are stepping into the realm of the timeless. You are leaping off your to-do list and plummeting into nondoing. You are surrendering into the space between breaths, out of which everything rises and passes away: your plans for the day, your child's laughter, the omelet you had for breakfast, the galaxies spiraling through space.

HOW TO JUST SIT THERE

Like all yogic arts, seated meditation is a process of touching the infinite by honoring the ordinary. Let's begin our journey this week by looking a little more closely at the basic body mechanics of the seated meditation posture.

Over the years, I've watched countless yogis use a meditation cushion as a kind of self-torture device. Hard-core yoga practitioners wrench their legs into full or half lotus for marathon sittings, apparently believing that bruising your inner thigh with your ankle is crucial to spiritual awakening. Seasoned meditators slump doggedly from one bell to the next, in lofty disregard for basic body mechanics, while wondering why they're spending yet another retreat focused primarily on the excruciating pain between their shoulder blades. People have told me that they can't meditate because they can't sit cross-legged on the floor.

It's not surprising that we can get so fixated on achieving the "perfect" meditation posture and then doggedly holding it even if it kills us. For most people, and particularly dedicated yoga practitioners, sitting cross-legged on a low cushion is synonymous with meditation. After all, have you ever seen an altar that featured a statue of the Buddha sitting in a chair?

For that reason I want to begin this week's practice—in which we'll focus primarily on going into seated-meditation posture and practices in more depth—with a liberating insight that may seem contradictory at first: you don't need a special posture to meditate, because meditation isn't a posture. It isn't even really something you *do*. It's a way of being that's relaxed and present, open to everything but chasing after nothing.

That said, it does help to have a formal method to cultivate that gentle, spacious attention. And it's useful to create an outer and inner environment in which to practice that method that grounds and relaxes the nervous system, sending signals to the primal brain that say, "It's safe. You can let down your guard." This is why so few ashrams are situated on a freeway meridian between a fire station and a discotheque. What you want is a meditation posture that's the equivalent of a creek-side temple in a quiet meadow, inviting you to settle in and relax awhile. And as you rest in that temple, the shy forest animals of your inner being—deer and raccoons, mountain lions and rattlesnakes—will reveal themselves as they emerge to drink.

For cultivating this silent inner witnessing, you need an asana that's *sthira* and *sukkha,* in the words of Patanjali's Yoga Sutra—a posture that's stable and comfortable that you can maintain for a significant amount of time without a lot of fidgeting, tension, or thinking about what to do next. You're probably not going to want to hang out in Headstand, Downward Dog, or a full back bend for 30 to 40 minutes at a stretch. And while lying down in Savasana is definitely stable and comfortable, there's a pretty high likelihood that you'll fall asleep if you do it for too long, especially if you've just eaten lunch.

So that's why sitting is so great—it's simple enough so you don't have to keep fussing over it. It's solid. It's restful. And if you doze off, eventually you'll start to fall forward and wake yourself up.

However, there's nothing magical about the cross-legged lotus pose that yogis are classically depicted in. In ancient India, chairs didn't exist: Everyone sat cross-legged on the ground or on low cushions, and so from early childhood, their hips and lower backs adapted to that position. By contrast, modern industrialized humans are generally plopped into car seats and high chairs from infancy, and by age six we're sitting at desks for a good part of the day. So while sitting cross-legged on a cushion may be comfortable for many people, please don't fret if it doesn't work for you.

What *is* important, if you're going to do formal meditation practice for any length of time, is the alignment of your head, neck, spine, and pelvis. A spine that's balanced and at ease supports the relaxation of your whole nervous system. Imbalances and misalignments of these major structures create tension and pain, sending alarm signals to your brain that in turn generate further anxiety. It's hard to soften and be present if your whole body is screaming *Emergency!* It's possible to open to pain through meditation, of course, to learn to be with it kindly as it arises and passes away. But why create it unnecessarily?

When the skull, rib cage, and pelvis are properly aligned, the cerebrospinal fluid can circulate freely, bathing and nourishing the brain and spinal cord as the craniosacral rhythms pulse unimpeded. In the language of the yogis, the prana—the life force—can flow with ease through the *sushumna nadi,* the central river of energy that courses through your core. The balanced alignment of the skeletal structure allows the musculature to relax so you're not tensing (subtly or not so subtly) just to stay upright. The diaphragm can widen and soften so the breath can billow through the whole body.

Seated Variations

A variety of different supported and unsupported sitting postures— basically just different arrangements of the hips, pelvis, and legs— facilitate this proper alignment of the spine and torso. In this chapter we'll explore three of them: the simple cross-legged position known in hatha yoga as Sukhasana (Easy Pose), a supported kneeling position that's a variation of the hatha yoga pose Virasana (Hero's Pose), and a chair-seated posture.

In your own sitting practice, feel free to choose whichever one works best for you—or to cycle through them regularly to ease repetitive stress on your body. Experiment with all of them though, so you become comfortable doing sitting meditation in a variety of postures. That way, when injury, illness, aging, or other physical changes require you to change the form of your practice, you'll be at ease with this alteration. It's a drag to have your spiritual well-being dependent upon, say, the cartilage in your knee.

And whichever form you choose, remember this important principle: Your meditation posture is not a yoga stretch. There are many wonderful asanas you can do to open your hips, pelvis, and shoulders and strengthen your core. However, your meditation pose should not be one of them. When you settle in to meditate for long periods of time, don't push your physical edge. To do so risks physical strain and injury and also undercuts the ease that nourishes meditative opening.

Basic Setups for Seated Meditation

Note that in all the following postures, the basic alignment of the head, neck, shoulders, and spine remains the same. You're looking for a way to sit where your spine can rest easily in its natural curves, with the skull balanced over the shoulder girdle and the shoulder girdle balanced over the pelvis. To maintain the natural curve of the lumbar spine, it's important to be able to tip your pelvis slightly forward, so you're sitting up on the front of your sitting bones, not slumping back.

The following instructions, therefore, focus on setting up the lower body as a base of support that facilitates this pelvic tilt and spinal alignment. Each of the three seated postures I describe share two common elements:

1. A solid base with the support of a cushion, chair, or ground. If parts of your lower body are floating untethered in space, you will feel unstable, setting your mind subtly—or not so subtly—on edge. So make sure, whatever posture you choose, that you have a wide and stable base, with the grounding of the sitting bones into your cushion or chair counterbalanced by the grounding of your feet or your knees on the earth.

2. An open angle between the torso and the thighs, so that the

creases of your groin creases—the seams where your thighs meet your torso—are soft and open. To achieve this, the knees should be slightly lower than the hip bones—this angle can be greater than 90 degrees but not less. This spaciousness in the groin creases allows the pelvis to tip slightly forward so you sit easily on the front of your sitting bones and the spine can be upright in its natural curves.

■ For a video primer on meditation posture, go to annecushman .com/practices.

Simple Cross-Legged Pose
(Sukhasana)

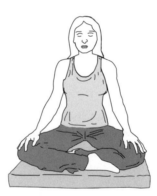

If you choose a cross-legged meditation posture, I recommend the one known to yogis as Sukhasana (Easy Pose), with one shin folded snugly in front of and parallel to the other. Alternate which leg is in front with every sitting so you don't create structural imbalances over time. Even if you are comfortable sitting flat on the floor, give yourself the support of a firm cushion under the sitting bones to encourage ease in the paraspinal muscles. Make sure you give yourself enough height that the knees can be lower than the hip bones.

If your knees bob in space, try adding an extra cushion. If your knees still float no matter how high you pile the cushions, check to see if your pelvis can tilt forward enough that you can sit on your sitting bones with the spine upright. If so, you can remain cross-legged, but add support—such as a folded blanket—under each knee. If the pelvis tips back so the spine is rounded, your hips are not yet open enough for the cross-legged position. If that's the case, try the Kneeling Meditation Pose (below).

I generally do not recommend full or half lotus—which for most people torques the knee. Even if you regularly practice full or half lotus in your yoga practice, beware of these asanas for long periods of meditation (more than 5 to 10 minutes at a time).

Even if you can get into these postures easily, the slow repetitive stress on the knee joint can cause injury over time.

Kneeling Meditation Pose

(Virasana or *Seiza*)

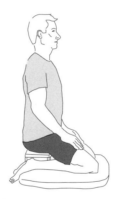

If the shape of your hip joints—or tightness in the muscles that surround them—prohibits you from comfortably sitting cross-legged, try kneeling instead. (This posture resembles the yoga pose Virasana or the Japanese seated position known as *seiza*—some people also refer to it as Burmese-style sitting.) Many meditation supply stores sell small wooden meditation benches specifically for this purpose (including folding travel benches). Or you can just turn your meditation cushion on its side and straddle it like a horse. (For most people, straddling a cushion without turning it on its side pushes the legs too wide for comfort.)

This kneeling position has several advantages. The knees will naturally be lower than the hips, creating an open angle in the groin and making it easy for the pelvis to tip into the proper angle. You'll also have a solid base of support, with the whole length of the shins and the top of the feet on the floor. Make sure you kneel on a padded surface so you don't create pain in the tender front of the knee. Some people find that the pressure on the tops of the feet creates pain in the ankles or arch. If that's the case for you, slide back so the knees and shins are supported by your padding (zabuton or folded blanket) but the feet and ankles drop off the back onto a lower pad such as a yoga mat.

Chair-Seated Pose

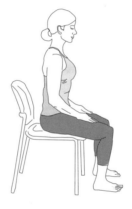

Sitting on a chair is a perfectly respectable posture for meditation. On long retreats, even seasoned meditators often cycle through periods of chair sitting to ease stress on knees, shoulders, and lower back. If you choose to sit in a chair, be sure to select one with a firm seat and upright back. Most chair seats slope slightly downward from front to back—exactly the opposite of the movement you want in the pelvis. If that's true for yours, level the seat by placing a pad or folded yoga mat on it.

Don't lean against the back of the chair. The chair is primarily to ease stress on the hips and knees and put the pelvis in the proper position—it's not meant as a backrest.

Instead, sit on your sitting bones toward the forward edge of your chair, with the feet flat on the ground. Now check the angle between your thighs and your torso. If it's less than 90 degrees—in other words, if your knees are higher than your hip joints—add more height beneath your buttocks. A folded yoga mat works great for this purpose. If your feet dangle, slip a pad or zafu beneath them.

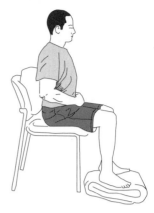

If you absolutely need support for your spine, don't lean backward to contact the back of the chair—again, this action tips the pelvis in the wrong direction, flattening the natural curve in the lumbar spine. Instead, try slipping a zafu on its side between your back and the chair back to support the spine while maintaining its lift.

Alignment of Upper Body in Seated Meditation

Once you've established your seat in one of these three positions—or any other seat of your choosing—tune in to the alignment of your upper body. Gently round and arch the lower back a few times, tilting the bowl of the pelvis forward and back until you're centered on your sitting bones. Sway front to back, then side to side, until you sense the skull balanced lightly over the pelvis. Your head weighs about twelve pounds, so if it migrates forward even slightly, over time its tug will contribute to the stabbing pain between the shoulder blades that longtime meditators know so well. If you're unsure, have a friend check your posture from the side: the centers of your ears should be aligned directly over the heads of your shoulders.

Whenever I find that I've been swept away by a tsunami of thoughts, I check my posture as I bring myself back to the present moment—often I find that my head has involuntarily craned forward, as if I were chasing the thoughts with my nose, like a dog trailing a rabbit through the underbrush.

Arrange your skeletal structure for maximum balance so that the bones hold themselves up with minimal muscular activity and your whole nervous system has the opportunity to release.

Meditators are sometimes instructed to "straighten their spine." But remember that the spinal column is not, in fact, straight. A healthy spine undulates through natural curves—drawing slightly inward at the neck (the cervical spine), outward through the region of the upper back (the thoracic spine), inward again through the lower back (lumbar spine), outward at the sacrum, and inward at the tailbone. So instead of straining to straighten your back, think of lengthening the spine upward as if being lifted from the crown of the head, while continuing to release your pelvis into the support of the earth. This allows the spine to relax into its natural curves around a central vertical axis. Slightly lower the chin and lift the back of the skull to create space at the base of the occiput, where the head meets the neck. This gesture slightly lowers your forebrain, which yogis say helps to "cool" the mind.

Rest your hands lightly on your thighs or knees. With palms down, you'll feel more grounded; with palms faceup, you'll feel more energized. Experiment to see what works best for you on any given day. Close your eyes or let your relaxed gaze rest on a point on the floor in front of you. Soften the gates of your senses—your inner ears, the root of your tongue, the muscles around your eyes.

Imagine a river of energy pouring down from the sky and through the crown of your head, through the center of your skull, through the center of your heart space, out the floor of your pelvis, and down into the earth. At the same time, this river of energy flows in the opposite direction: up from the center of the earth, through your body, and out the crown of the head. Let your body make whatever micromovements it needs to align itself around this central column, finding its own ever-shifting balance.

Just as you've been practicing over the last few weeks, invite your body to receive the breath so your sitting posture is alert but relaxed.

Coping with Common Meditator Pains

Hold any position for 30 to 40 minutes and a certain amount of discomfort is inevitable. Structural imbalances and long-held tension will naturally begin to reveal themselves—and it may not be pleasant. One of the arts of meditation is learning to be with uncomfortable sensations without reflexively bolting (we'll work with this in more depth in week 8). However, there's no need to create pain unnecessarily. And it's important to learn to distinguish between garden-variety restlessness and discomfort that you can learn to be with patiently and urgent warning signals from the body.

With that in mind, here are a few common meditation complaints you may run into:

Knee pain. Growing up in a culture where sitting in chairs is the norm, many people have hips that don't easily rotate externally. To compensate for the limitations in the hip joint, in order to achieve a cross-legged seat, practitioners may torque their knee so the lower shin is no longer aligned with the upper thigh bone. This position may feel fine at first, but by the end of a sitting your knee may feel like someone is pounding it with a jackhammer. Warning: Do not persist at sitting cross-legged with a sharp stabbing pain in your knee—you can cause long-term damage to the joint. Change to a chair or a bench instead.

If the shin and thigh are correctly aligned but the knee still feels compressed, try relieving it by slipping a slim padding—such as a folded washcloth—into the back of the knee joint. Again, if this doesn't work, change positions.

Pain between the shoulder blades. First check the alignment of your head. Each inch that the skull migrates forward from center alignment adds an additional ten pounds of weight for your neck and upper back to carry. Try gliding it back into alignment. Also, make sure you are allowing the spine to rock slightly with the breath, as you practiced in week 3 (practice 3.16 on page 84). Gripping the paraspinal muscles creates rigidity and pain in the upper thoracic area. By contrast, subtle micromovements in response to the breath will continually release tension and create ease in the whole body.

Neck and shoulder tension. Are your trapezius muscles—those wide bands on either side of the neck—turning into iron rods? Try raising the support of your hands by draping a folded blanket across your knees or resting your hands at the center line of your body on a zafu turned on its side in your lap or between your legs. Many people find that unburdening the neck and shoulders from the weight of the arms brings more ease to their sitting posture.

Once you settle in and feel reasonably comfortable, resist fidgeting. If your posture becomes so uncomfortable that it's consuming all of your attention, you can mindfully readjust. I once heard a meditator ask Thich Nhat Hanh, "Shouldn't I use pain in my meditation posture as an opportunity to practice being with suffering?" With a gentle smile, Thich Nhat Hanh asked in return, "Don't you have enough suffering in your life you can practice with? Do you need to create it through your meditation?"

Now What? Cultivating Focus

So you've gotten yourself seated on your cushion or chair or bench or yoga bolster. You've tweaked every detail of your posture. You've staked out a meditation campsite with all of your essential gear: cushions, bench, chair, zabuton, shawl, water bottle, candle, Buddha statue—perhaps some crampons and a compass and an ice ax, because you just never know what might happen. Now what?

Like any yoga, seated meditation is an intersection of at least two things: what you're doing with your body and where you're placing your attention. There are hundreds of wonderful practices that you can do while you're sitting in meditation, from mantra recitation and candle gazing to loving-kindness and breath concentration.

Nearly all of these practices fall into one of three categories:

Concentration practices collect and unify the heart and mind so you can focus your attention without distractions.

Mindfulness practices open to and investigate—with nonjudgmental, loving awareness—the nature of whatever is rising and passing away inside or around you.

Heart practices systematically cultivate qualities such as kindness, joy, compassion, generosity, and equanimity.

These are not strictly separate categories—each one contains elements of all the others. When you practice meditation, you will always rely on concentration and mindfulness working together, infused with heart. It takes a certain amount of collecting and unifying the heart and mind to be able to practice mindfulness. Mindfulness practice, directed and sustained over time on the same object, becomes deeper concentration. And to be effective, both of these practices need to be infused with such qualities as kindness and compassion—which, in turn, are supported by and spontaneously arise from mindful presence. The art of meditation involves balancing all of these elements—adding the appropriate seasoning to your meditative broth according to what flavor you want to accent.

In a daily meditation session, for example, you might begin with a short mindfulness check-in—scanning your body, heart, and mind to see how you are in this moment and what you're bringing to your practice today. (For an example of such a practice, see Checking In with Body, Heart, and Mind, page 130.)

Then you might settle into some form of concentration practice to gather and unify the scattered, flying specks of your attention so you can be more fully present moment to moment. For example, you might do a body-sensing scan or use your breath as the anchor to which you return your attention again and again.

Once your attention has become relatively stable, you have a choice: to emphasize concentration or to emphasize mindfulness. To strengthen your concentration, you would come back again and again to the same focus—such as the sensation of breath at a specific part of the body or a systematic body scan such as you were introduced to in week 1 (Exploring the Whole Body). To emphasize mindfulness, you would keep the lens of your attention wider, just noticing whatever was arising within the field of your awareness.

When we first begin practicing meditation, our minds are generally so scattered that for most people it is useful to cultivate our capacity to return again and again to the same object. If we try to practice pure mindfulness, we are too easily swept away and get lost in the contents of our experience. In the context of a long, silent retreat, this sustained concentration practice for many hours a day can move the meditator into deep states of blissful absorption (known in Pali as *jhana* and in Sanskrit as *dhyana*—the seventh limb of Patanjali's classical eight-limbed yoga system).

As you recall from chapter 2, the Buddha practiced very deep forms of concentration meditation with the greatest yogis of his day.

However, he discovered something very important: that these bliss states left untouched the deep patterns of action and thought that lead to suffering. Many a meditator has returned home from an intensive retreat and found herself embroiled within minutes in a fight with her partner. The Buddha found it was more useful to take this focused attention and use it to investigate the true nature of our embodied human lives. This is the practice of mindfulness. To practice mindfulness, you don't need deep states of absorption. You just need a mind that's collected enough that you can show up for your experience—and notice when you're not there.

And from this stable place it's possible to deliberately cultivate qualities of the heart such as joy and peace that can radiate not just through your meditation practice but through all of your life.

FROM FAKING IT TO MAKING IT ⤳ Kate Johnson

Kate Johnson teaches yoga in New York City schools.

In my yoga teacher training, we were supposed to keep a meditation journal and meditate ten minutes a day for a month. I totally faked the journal. I didn't meditate at all and made up the whole journal the day before it was due: "Day One—Sat 10 minutes. Felt really calm. . . ."

I had this resistance to the idea of doing nothing. I was a professional dancer. My mind couldn't be quiet unless I was moving. My approach was to become really absorbed in movement or do a lot of movement to tire myself out so I was too tired to think. It was all about controlling my experience. I didn't want to sit down and check out my experience and just be with it.

Then, about four months after my teacher training, I fell through a trapdoor in a restaurant. I tore the ACL ligament in my knee and crushed my left hand. I needed three surgeries. I wasn't able to use my left hand for three months, and I was on crutches for almost a year. I was bored, I was in pain, and I didn't know if I would ever be able to dance again.

So I got really interested in this idea of meditation as a way to work with what I had avoided before. So many things were beyond my control. Here was a practice that could help me bear this lack of control.

I didn't realize how much energy I'd been putting into resisting my actual experience. It was a relief to be able to let go of that struggle and open up to what was actually going on without trying to make something else happen. I had been so afraid of doing that.

Through the various surgeries and physical therapy, I got meditation instructions for working with the physical pain I was dealing with. I began to notice it wasn't always present in the same way. It came in waves: there would be periods where the pain was building up, then a peak, then it would subside. So when it got bad, I no longer had the sense that it would be like this forever. I was able to go to that place in my body that didn't hurt for a while, that wasn't in pain. As a professional dancer, I had a lot of fear about my future. Meditation helped me to be able to be with that process of recovery without knowing how it would come out, to be with that uncertainty.

Now I teach yoga full-time in public high schools in New York. My students are almost all students of color, black and Latino, mostly low income. Many of them have experienced a lot of trauma—the trauma of being poor in the United States, racism, or physical abuse. My meditation practice has made teaching in this situation more sustainable. The average turnover for teachers is five years—they just get burned out. My meditation practice has helped me roll with the punches a little bit. I feel that my meditation practice is kind of like a balm, like putting lotion on my dry, itchy nerves. It helps me feel flexible and a little more spacious. I can be a stable presence, so students know that I am going to react in predictable ways to what they give me. I feel calmer. Anything can happen, and everything's going to be okay.

WEEK 5 PRACTICES

Practice 5.30:   Seated Meditation—Sensing the Breath
(30–40 minutes)   133

This week, set aside at least 30 minutes each day for seated meditation. Precede it with as much asana and pranayama as you have time
for—ideally, at least 30 minutes—to allow yourself to experience how
the practices mutually support and deepen one another.

As in weeks 1–4, your meditation instructions for this week will
continue to emphasize collecting and unifying your mind by drawing
your attention back again and again to the anchor of your breath and
body. In subsequent weeks, you will begin to widen the lens of your
attention to include mindfulness of other aspects of your experience,
such as feelings and states of mind.

Begin each meditation session with Checking In with Body, Heart,
and Mind (below). Then follow it with either Seated Meditation—Body
Scan (page 131) or Seated Meditation—Sensing the Breath (page 133).

If you choose the body-sensing meditation for that day's practice, emphasize body sensing in your asana, using some of the practices from
weeks 1 and 2. If you choose the breath-sensing meditation practice, focus
on the breath in your asana, using the practices from weeks 3 and 4.

After day 3 settle on one practice or the other for the rest of the
week so you can deepen into it.

PRACTICE 5.28
Checking In with Body, Heart, and Mind (5–10 minutes)

*Begin each sitting period by welcoming yourself home, as if greeting a dear
friend. Ask yourself:* How am I? *Then wait to feel the answer.*

First, check in with your body: Are you achy? Itchy? Bubbling with
sexual energy? Does your neck hurt from sitting at the computer too
long? Are you still digesting last night's enchiladas? Inquire with
friendly curiosity—not judging but befriending. See if there's any part
of your body that's calling for more tenderness.

See whether there's anywhere you can let go—a gripping in the
jaw or behind the eyes or in the lower belly. Is there anywhere you are

bracing your body against the natural wave of the breath? As you soften into connection with each part of your body, see if the breath responds by growing a little deeper.

Now check in with your emotions. You may find that it helps to put one hand on your heart and another on your belly, letting your hands become the physical expression of your kind attention. What's the emotional weather? Are storm clouds brewing or are the skies blue? Does a fog of loneliness hang over your inner hills? Don't get drawn into the fascinating story of why you're so mad or sad or excited. Instead, just let yourself feel the feelings themselves.

And now check in with your thoughts, the endless narration of opinions and plans and memories and comments that you may believe is telling you the truth about who you really are. Is the broadcast rapid and loud? Or relatively subdued? Are you filled with plans for your day? Or are you doing the instant replay of what just happened? Have compassion for your busy, scheming mind—working so tirelessly, if misguidedly, to keep you safe.

Finally, align yourself with your deepest intention for your practice today, whatever it may be: perhaps to be present with an open heart for whatever arises or to use whatever practice you have chosen as a tool to help you wake up—returning to it, again and again, with loving determination whenever you drift away.

Once you have completed your check-in, move seamlessly into either of the next two practices: 5.29 (Body Scan) or 5.30 (Sensing the Breath).

PRACTICE 5.29
Seated Meditation—Body Scan (30–40 minutes)

Once you've checked in and set your intention for your practice, invite yourself on an inner journey through the terrain of your body.

This practice isn't dramatically different from the reclining body scan in week 1 (Exploring the Whole Body, on page 44). But it is a deepening of it, especially if you are not accustomed to doing longer periods of sitting meditation. Sitting upright, you're less likely to fall asleep or drift down a river of daydreams. Also, you're more likely to encounter a whole armada of strong—

and potentially uncomfortable—sensations as you stay in this position for a sustained period. This is actually a gift, believe it or not. Learning to work with sensations in a meditative way is a foundational skill in your practice, which we'll build on as we move through the weeks ahead.

From your explorations in previous weeks, you are familiar with this inner journey. (If you need a refresher, visit Exploring the Whole Body.) So take your time and let yourself enjoy it. There is nowhere else your attention needs to bustle off to.

As you travel through your body with your attention, notice the areas you tend to rush through or skip over. When teachers give guided instructions for this practice, they often skip the genitals so as not to provoke discomfort in a public class. But this is your practice. You are invited to feel every part of your body, even the parts you might normally neglect.

Sometimes it's helpful to focus your attention with words: *Jaw. Tongue. Thigh. Big toe.* But remember, you are not *visualizing* that part of the body. You are feeling it directly, from the inside. If you find an area of strong sensation, linger there awhile, getting curious: Is this prickling? Tingling? Burning? Is it solid or changing? When you find areas of tension, invite them to soften, but don't demand that they do.

When you find an area where there is very little sensation, linger there and see if it wants to speak to you any further. But don't get lost in stories about why it may be silent.

When you notice that your mind has drifted off—as it will—don't be hard on yourself. Instead, appreciate the fact that now you're back. If it helps, name what took you away: *Thinking. Sleeping. Planning.* Include it in your kind awareness. Scan your body to see whether your thought journey left a trail of tension behind, and if so, encourage it to soften. Then invite yourself back to the last place you remember inhabiting and fully reinhabit it before continuing on your journey.

When you have completed a pass through your body, reverse directions and head toward the crown of your head again. This reversal is an interesting moment. You may feel that you have already made this trip. Why tramp back and forth over the same familiar pathway? Make the choice to continue to deepen inward. Often, in hatha yoga, we stay interested in our body by constantly creating new sensations through increasingly varied and challenging movements. But in seated meditation, we learn to feel more not by creating stronger sensations but by increasing our sensitivity—by opening on deeper and deeper levels to what we may have imagined we already knew.

So keep traversing the terrain. There is nowhere to get—once you get to your toes, you know you will just turn around again. So slow down and let more and more be revealed.

As someone who prides yourself on an active asana practice, you may be amazed to discover how difficult it can be to hold this relatively simple asana for a long period of time. You may get to know your body in a way that you haven't in years of advanced asanas. Structural imbalances may become glaringly apparent. Areas of unconscious holding may scream for your attention.

In your yoga practice, you may have gotten very good at avoiding any uncomfortable sensations. Sure, there may be asanas that you don't like, but you can always skip them or flow in and out of them. But in sitting meditation, there's no escape.

Or perhaps you'll encounter blissful feelings—subtle pockets of pleasure that expand into ecstasy in the warmth of your attention. Try not to flinch away from the uncomfortable areas or try to fix them; don't try to prolong the delicious ones. Just continue your careful exploration.

When you hold the body as the object of meditation, the distinction between body and mind gradually breaks down. Is it the mind that is aware of the body? Is the body aware of itself? Or is the body aware of the mind?

When the bell rings, don't drop the practice immediately. Notice where your attention is resting. Then let it expand to hold the whole field of your body—its sensations flickering like a billion candles in the vast space of your awareness.

PRACTICE 5.30
Seated Meditation—Sensing the Breath (30–40 minutes)

Like practice 5.29, this one flows naturally from practice 5.28: Checking In with Body, Heart, and Mind (page 130).

After you have done your check-in and set your intention, let your attention be naturally magnetized to the feeling of your breath coming and going—which you've become sensitized to in your explorations in weeks 3 and 4.

If you're feeling agitated, you may want to spend a few minutes lengthening the pause after the exhalation and/or lengthening the exhalation itself. If you're feeling sluggish and sleepy, practice lengthening the inhalation and/or the pause after the inhalation.

Then let go of controlling the breath and simply receive it. Observe where you experience the breath most strongly. Let your attention naturally settle around that area.

For a body-centered breath meditation that organically ties in to an asana practice, it's best not to choose the nostrils as a place of focus, as this focal point tends to draw the attention into the head. Instead, choose somewhere lower in the body. Here are a few options:

- The gentle swelling and releasing of the belly as the diaphragm moves down and up. See if you can sense the movement not just in the front of the body but expanding in all directions— widening to the sides, expanding into the lower back and kidneys. Sense the breath as energy radiating beyond the confines of your skin.
- The movement of the diaphragm up and down in synchrony with the broadening and releasing of the pelvic floor and perineum.
- The release of the rib cage as the rim of the diaphragm expands and contracts.
- The whole body moving with the breath as you hold it in the wide lens of your attention—skin softening, belly pulsing, collarbones broadening, heads of the shoulders widening and retracting.

Wherever you rest your attention, keep a relaxed openness to the pulsation of breath. Don't strain to "follow" the breath. Instead, receive each breath with open arms.

As you practiced in weeks 3 and 4, keep the body fluid. Don't freeze into rigor mortis meditation. Remember that the diaphragm is attached to the spine as well as the rib cage, so each breath in and out ripples along the whole length of the spinal column.

If you find yourself hardening, take a couple of breaths to relax the paraspinal muscles by slightly tucking the tailbone and rounding the upper back as you exhale and draw the belly back, dropping the chin toward the breastbone. Then, as you inhale, roll the spine open again like an unfurling fern, from the tip of the tailbone up to the crown of the head.

Be very kind to yourself. Your attention will wander from your breath a thousand times over the course of your meditation period. You are not a stern disciplinarian chasing down your truant attention and dragging it back to your breath by its hair. You are welcoming yourself home, again and again. Your thinking mind is doing its best, earnestly scurrying around trying to keep you safe. It has been rewarded for doing so over and over again throughout your life. So bow to it. Thank it for its efforts. And then relax back into the whole-body caress of your breath.

As you return to your breath, check in with your body. Has it clenched? Has your head migrated forward? Have your eyes hardened and your shoulders climbed toward your ears? This is an important moment. By softening your musculature, you are sending a message of ease throughout your whole nervous system, physically manifesting kindness toward yourself. By realigning your skeletal structure, you are realigning yourself with your intention to be present.

Pay particular attention to the spaces between the breaths—the empty pause after the exhale, the full pause after the inhale. Allow yourself to surrender into these spaces as the breath emerges from stillness and empties back into stillness again.

When the bell rings for the end of your meditation period, if you have been pulled out to sea by a riptide of thinking, swim back to the refuge of breath. Receive a few conscious breaths before releasing from your meditation posture.

Poses to Prepare for Seated Meditation—and to Release Tension Afterward

All hatha yoga asanas prepare you for meditation; that is, after all, what they were designed for. However, a few specific poses are especially useful for helping prepare for your sitting practice or discharge any tension you may have accumulated afterward. Whatever poses you choose, practice them with sensitivity as a mindfulness meditation in themselves.

Spine. If you have only a few minutes to practice asanas before you sit, focus on increasing flexibility in your spine. Open the spine in all directions: Flex and extend it from front to back (say, in the familiar Cat-Cow or flowing from Upward to Downward Dog). Open it laterally through simple side bends. Rotate it through seated or side-lying twists. These movements are also blissful to do *after* sitting meditation. Remember to respect the delicacy of the spine—stay well within your natural range of motion.

Hips and knees. If you aspire to sit cross-legged on a cushion to meditate, it helps to have hips that easily rotate externally so your knees can stay in proper alignment. Some classic hip openers include Pigeon and Bound Angle (Baddha Konasana) and standing poses such as Triangle and Warrior II.

Neck and shoulders. With the arms in Gomukhasana (Cow Face Pose), glide the elbows up and down and from side to side (this is another delicious one for unwinding after you sit). Energize and release through Downward Dog and Dolphin Pose (a Dog variation with the forearms on the floor and the hands clasped). Or roll in and out of Bridge Pose or release the neck in the other direction through Plow.

Lower back. Keep your sittings juicy and energized by maintaining mobility in your lower back and sacrum. Especially useful are back bends such as Cobra Pose and Locust Pose, which strengthen and tone the lower back while increasing flexibility. If you don't have a lower-back injury, balance these with Seated Forward Bends that tip the sacrum in the opposite direction.

Upper back. Help correct the forward head position that can cause upper-back problems by practicing Nose Nod: lie flat on your back and, without flattening your neck, move the tip of your nose in the direction of your sternum, then back up again. Open the heart area through supported back bends over a block or bolster.

In Your Daily Life This Week

This week, in addition to your longer sitting-meditation practice, try sprinkling 5-minute meditation breaks throughout your day. Arrived early at your dentist appointment? Meditate in the car for 5 minutes instead of going in. Finished answering your e-mail? Instead of plunging into the next task, sit for 5 minutes at your desk. Do a 3-minute check-in with body, emotions, and thoughts, then gather your attention on your breath for 2 minutes.

You'll be amazed what a difference these minimeditations can make, especially if you've started your day with a formal sitting. It's like brewing yourself a big pot of peppermint tea first thing in the morning, then taking sips of it throughout your day.

RESOURCES

There are countless excellent meditation books available in multiple Buddhist and non-Buddhist traditions. A good primer for the mindfulness meditation we're practicing in this program is Sharon Salzberg's *Real Happiness: The Power of Meditation.* Or for a different flavor, try Thich Nhat Hanh's classic *The Miracle of Mindfulness.* The Buddhist yoga teacher Jill Satterfield has been integrating meditation in motion for almost thirty years; check her out at vajrayoga.com.

Exploring Standing and Walking Meditation

A COUPLE OF YEARS AGO, in the middle of a weeklong meditation retreat, I slipped and fell down the stairs outside my dorm.

I had paused in the pale dawn mist to put on my shoes, watching a doe graze with her fawn and three turkeys strut down the path to the meditation hall. Wrapping my shawl around my head, I felt noble and serene, like the star of a documentary about mindfulness. Then I stepped onto the wooden stairs, slick with half-frozen dew—and my feet skidded out from under me. I fell on my rear, bouncing *boom-boom-boom* all the way down the steps like a cartoon character and landing with a yelp at the bottom. All around me, yogis had paused on their way to meditation and were gazing at me in silent alarm, as were the deer and the turkeys. I waved and grimaced sheepishly, and then gingerly picked myself up—no longer feeling like a mindfulness movie star—and hobbled off to meditation.

There I quickly discovered that when you've just bounced down a flight of stairs on your butt, the last place you want to be is at an event where every other item on the daily schedule is "sitting." An emergency trip to my chiropractor revealed that I had a fractured tailbone—and that the only thing I could do to help it get better was to stay off it as much as possible. So rather than bail out on the retreat—or on my meditation practice for the next six months or so—I decided to take the opportunity to go more deeply into the practices of standing and walking meditation.

Standing and walking are two of the four classic meditation modalities mentioned by the Buddha—the others being sitting and lying down, both of which we've already dived into in some depth in this program.

In hatha yoga, the standing posture known as Tadasana (Mountain Pose) or Samasthiti is the foundation for all the other, more-elaborate standing postures. But in most yoga classes, we rarely hold Tadasana for more than a couple of minutes before going on to other—and presumably more important—standing postures or vinyasa flows. And in most meditation circles, sitting is generally viewed—implicitly if not explicitly—as the superior path, so much so that the words *meditation* and *sitting* are often used interchangeably.

And while meditation retreats generally alternate periods of sitting and walking throughout the day, yoga practitioners often view a walking meditation period as the perfect opportunity to—you guessed it!—do a little asana. Slowly walking back and forth over the same thirty-foot section of ground may not seem to cut it when your body is longing for back bends, shoulder stands, and twists.

But as I remembered during my forced abstinence from sitting meditation, both standing and walking meditation are deep practices, with distinctive benefits and challenges. This week we're going to explore the ways that these two practices can work in concert with yoga asanas and seated meditation to both deepen your mindfulness practice and broaden it into your life in new ways.

NOT JUST STANDING AROUND

Before I fractured my tailbone, I thought of standing meditation merely as a backup option to use on a long retreat if I were too sleepy or physically uncomfortable to sit. It was a public admission of meditative failure: "I can't handle the sitting, so why don't I try standing for a while?"

But as it turned out, that's like thinking "Tylenol isn't doing the trick, so why don't I take a little LSD instead?" As I quickly realized, standing meditation is a potent practice in its own right, with dramatic and unique effects on the body, mind, and nervous system. It's as stable as sitting meditation, and as you build up the strength for it, it can be practiced for equally long periods of time. And it offers a powerful feeling of grounded connection down through the feet and legs into the earth.

When I introduce standing meditation on yoga retreats, some yogis always resist it at first. As hatha yogis we tend to love the more dramatic and vigorous standing poses—the two Warrior, Half Moon, Dancer's, and Tree. But holding a simple standing position more than five minutes can seem pretty boring—after all, we're just standing there! To an achievement-oriented yogi, standing doesn't offer either the contemplative cachet of seated meditation or the workout of a Warrior sequence.

But overcome your initial skepticism and you'll find this practice both rewarding and challenging. It seems such a simple gesture— what could be more basic than to be a human being standing upright? But just as with sitting practice, if you stand in meditation for more than ten or fifteen minutes, a host of long-held—and probably largely unconscious—physical and energetic patterns of misalignment and contraction will begin to announce themselves. They may manifest as aching shoulders, a tight neck, a fog of exhaustion, or just the over-powering restless desire to get moving. Some of these may be familiar to you from your sitting practice, but others are likely to be whole new somatic revelations. They might be accompanied by strong emotions such as anger or agitation. You may feel an intensified awareness of places where the flow of energy feels blocked—particularly in and through the hip joints and inner groin creases, the junctures of the energetic superhighways that run through the pelvis to connect the upper and lower bodies. As these patterns begin to unwind, you may tremble, tingle, and sweat. You may feel waves of intense pleasure or almost unbearable boredom.

And if you persist in your practice, the qualities of groundedness and relaxation you cultivate through standing meditation practice will directly enhance both your seated meditation and your asana practice—not to mention your life.

While the basic standing-meditation posture is very like the yoga pose Tadasana, it differs in some respects from the way Tadasana is typically taught. Unlike the usual yoga-class Tadasana, standing meditation is designed to be practiced for long periods of time—so the muscles need to be dynamically relaxed rather than forcefully engaged. You aren't standing like a soldier, preparing to conquer your body and mind. You're standing like a weathered oak—your roots tunneling deep for underground springs, owls nesting in your branches, squirrels feasting on your acorns.

GOING NOWHERE: THE BASICS OF WALKING MEDITATION

When my son was three, we used to walk every day to a park a few blocks away. A neighbor's dog would always join us—an ancient, fat, smelly, waddling, and almost-blind beagle named Tony, whom Skye adored. We'd often take more than an hour to get to our destination—Skye enraptured by wild onions and blackberry brambles and mysterious bits of plastic; Tony enraptured by endless things to smell and/or pee on. Sometimes I'd catch myself trying to rush them along: *Gotta get to the park! We've got swings to swing on! Sand to put in buckets! Graham crackers to eat!* When I remembered to treat the outing as walking meditation, I was able to forget the destination and surrender to the journey. Now, looking back, those leisurely ambles shimmer in my memory as some of the most precious moments of Skye's toddler-hood.

Walking meditation is a chance to be present in your body for the ordinary human miracle of walking on the earth. It gives you the chance to cultivate embodied presence while moving through a very simple and ordinary activity. You're not break dancing. You're not doing a drop back from a headstand into a back bend. You're just putting one foot in front of the other, as you've been doing since you were a year old.

What distinguishes walking meditation from ordinary walking is that you're not trying to get anywhere. Usually you're walking *to* something—the refrigerator, the post office, the top of a windswept ridge. But in walking meditation the destination is the walking itself. On the walking-meditation paths at Plum Village, Thich Nhat Hanh's retreat center in France, a sign is posted: "You have already arrived."

Like any meditation form, walking meditation supports the cultivation of both concentration and mindfulness. But walking meditation has a few distinct features. Since it's a moving meditation, it can brighten your energy when you're feeling sleepy and release discomfort that may have built up in more static postures. Of course, asana practice can do this as well. But because the forms of asana are more complex, they're more likely to draw you into mental activity and project orientation. And walking meditation is a highly portable practice that you can use throughout your day: walking into the kitchen to get a cup of tea, walking the dog around the block. No one will even know you're doing it, whereas if you try a vinyasa flow from your car into the bank, you're sure to attract a couple of curious looks, even in California.

I'll offer you two variations of walking meditation to explore this week. The first is a more formal variation from the vipassana tradition, in which you'll walk back and forth over the same small area. The second is the more informal approach I learned from Thich Nhat Hanh, which looks a lot more like just taking a walk, but slower. See which one serves you better. Either way, I suggest that you precede your walking with a short period of standing meditation—at least 10 minutes. It's likely to dramatically increase your connection with your feet and the earth.

To make sure you have enough time for walking this week, you are welcome to substitute it for sitting meditation. Or if you're up for living dangerously, you can substitute walking for your asana practice and keep your seated meditation. Think of walking as just a very slow vinyasa between very simple yoga poses. How does that change the way you look at it?

THE YOGA OF WALKING   Stefan Zijlstra

Stefan Zijlstra is the owner of the Snow Buddha yoga studio in Anchorage, Alaska.

I run a company that cleans up after dogs. Now I have employees, but in the beginning I used to do the work myself. I would walk around and clean up after the dogs as walking meditation. I would notice when my mind wandered off and took me with it—and when I was just right there, bending over, cleaning up.

If you just think about this job, you'd think I wouldn't like it—but it's a great job once you get over the gross-out factor. It was very meditative work—outside all day, walking in different people's yards, with dogs around to play with. I was meditating with all of my senses, because the work involved seeing, touching, and, of course, also smelling.

Now I teach walking meditation a lot in my yoga classes. I have people just walk up and down their mats. Yoga and walking meditation are really similar. In both of them, it's not really about the form—it's just about training the awareness and the nonjudgmental attitude toward what's in the body and the mind. You're really starting to move into the fine details of awareness. If you're really zooming in on the details of walking—lifting, moving, placing, shifting—walking is a yoga pose in itself.

WEEK 6 PRACTICES

This week, please substitute Standing Meditation for part of your daily seated meditation, leaving the total meditation practice time the same as last week: 30 to 40 minutes each day. I suggest that you begin with a relatively short standing session—say, 5 minutes—and then move directly into seated meditation for the remainder of your meditation. Gradually increase the time until you are able to stand for 20 minutes or more. As with sitting meditation, you may find it easier to practice standing meditation after your asana practice, when the body is more open, energized, and relaxed. However, it's also interesting to do a period of standing meditation before your asana practice and see how that affects the quality of your yoga.

If your climate and neighborhood allow it, try doing the Standing Meditation practice outdoors with your bare feet directly on the earth (not on cement or even on wooden decking). Having the skin of your feet plugged in to naked soil, sand, or grass creates a wonderful sensation of sensual aliveness. But if you can't do this, just sense your energy body sending its roots down through carpet, floor, and cement foundations into the earth that's always there to meet it.

PRACTICE 6.31
Standing Meditation (10–30 minutes)

◀◎ For a guided audio version of standing meditation, go to www.shambhala.com/movingintomeditation.

As with seated meditation, the standing-meditation posture can be the foundation of many different kinds of practice. Anything you can practice seated you can practice standing—body scan, breath awareness, heart practices, mindfulness of any of the different levels of your multidimensional body. You may wish to use standing meditation to explore any of the practices we did last week—Checking In with Body, Heart, and Mind (page 130), Body Scan (page 131), and Sensing the Breath (page 133). As always, whichever you choose, stay with it for the duration of your practice to see how it affects you and what it reveals.

Come into a basic standing position with the feet about hip width apart. To begin with, let your attention drop into the soles of your feet, inviting them to be as sensitive as hands as they caress the earth. Roll around on your feet a bit, flexing and rolling over your toes, then picking up and replacing first one foot, then the other, like a cat kneading a blanket. Shift your weight from one foot to the other until the weight feels evenly divided. Rock your weight forward and back until you feel balanced directly over the midpoint of the arch. Lift your toes, pressing into the balls of the feet downward, and spread the toes wide, then see if you can place them back down one toe at a time. If you were standing on damp sand, would the impression made by the two feet be the same? Or would one footprint be deeper, clearer, or wider?

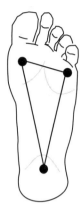

Feel into the triangle formed by the ball of the big toe, the ball of the little toe, and the midpoint of the heel. Can you spread your weight evenly among these points? Visualize the arches of the feet lifting like two halves of a divided dome, echoing the dome of the perineum, the dome of the diaphragm, and the dome of the soft palate—as if a stream of energy had fountained upward from the center of the earth to lift all four. Sense into the energy gateway located along the center line of the foot where the ball of the foot meets the arch, just inside and to the center of the ball of the foot—known in Chinese medicine as "bubbling well" and in yoga anatomy as *pada* chakra, the foot chakra. Notice whether your weight tends to collapse in toward the ankles or sprawl out.

Relax the soles of the feet, opening the energy gateways to the earth. Spend plenty of time here—remember, you're not running off anywhere anytime soon.

Now flow your attention gradually up the legs. Encourage the knees to be open, not locked, with a slight, externally imperceptible microbend to avoid hyperextending. Unlike in a formal Tadasana, don't engage the quadriceps to lift the kneecaps—this action will be too tiring over a lengthy hold. Instead, allow the quadriceps to rest in dynamic relaxation, naturally activating only as needed to maintain a balanced alignment.

Travel your attention up to the pelvis and release any gripping through the groins. Release your tailbone down toward the earth as if you had an actual tail anchoring you. If you have a hard time feeling this release, slightly bend the knees, then gradually let them straighten, as if eyes were opening at the backs of your knee creases. Relax any contraction of the perineum. Ask the breath to move fully into the belly, lower back, and kidney area.

Let the shoulders be relaxed and the chest open without throwing the chest forward and shoulders back in a military stance. Open your arms slightly away from the sides of your body, then relax them back down as if you had pillows of air in your armpits. Soften the jaws and the eyes, relaxing the gaze and opening the peripheral vision. Sense the balanced alignment of the skull over the pelvis and the pelvis over the feet. Feel a window of energy opening where the base of the skull meets the neck, as the occiput delicately lifts.

Now, just as you did when finding your seated-meditation alignment, imagine a river of energy pouring down from the sky. It flows through the crown of your head; down through the center of your skull, heart, and lower belly; and through your perineum down into the very center of the earth. At the same time, energy is flowing up from the core of the earth, lifting the arches of your feet and fountaining up through your pelvic floor, lower belly, and heart, and out through the crown of your head.

Let your skeletal structure find its own natural—and subtly ever-shifting—alignment around this central energetic axis. If you relax around it, your body will continually make whatever microadjustments are needed to stay in balance. This will be much more effective than constantly micromanaging the situation from your mind: *Okay, now draw the skull back. . . . Oops, no, now tip the pelvis forward. . . .* The natural curves of the spine oscillate around this energetic plumb line.

Once you have found your alignment, relax into spacious, full-body awareness.

Standing meditation seems particularly suited for body awareness with a wide lens—letting your attention hold the whole body and receive whatever presents itself most vividly. For most people, sensations in the feet, legs, and hips become particularly vivid. Let them emerge into the foreground of your attention. You may sense energy roots extending from the soles of the feet down into the earth. If other sensations become more intense, let your attention track them. As with any meditation practice, you're likely to get drawn off into plans, memories, and mental commentary. If this happens—or if you get overwhelmed by the myriad of sensations you're experiencing—bring your attention back to your lower legs and feet and to the feeling of contact between feet and ground.

When you've completed your standing meditation, move directly into sitting for the duration of your meditation period. Maintain a seamless flow of presence through the transition between postures. As you continue your meditation in the sitting position, notice any subtle—or not so subtle—differences in the quality and focus of your attention.

PRACTICE 6.32
Walking Meditation I (15–30 minutes)

If possible, do your walking meditation outside to enhance your connection with the earth, the sky, and the elements. However, if it's too rainy, snowy, or hot to be out, or if your neighborhood isn't conducive to meditation, it's fine to practice inside. Find a pathway about thirty to forty feet long; if you're inside, you may need to settle for something shorter. Make sure the ground is clear enough that you don't have to be constantly concerned about dodging puddles, climbing over rocks, or skirting around furniture.

The outward form of the practice is simple—all you're going to do is walk to the end of your chosen path, pause, turn around, pause again, and walk back. Then you're going to repeat this simple walking vinyasa over and over for the duration of the meditation period. However, within this simple form, a world of sensate aliveness awaits you—as well as infinite ways to vary the focus and quality of your attention.

Begin by spending a few minutes in standing meditation to connect with your body—and particularly with the grounding of your feet and legs into the earth. Then begin to move at the speed that keeps you most intimately connected with your body sensations and gives you the greatest sense of ease. Usually, this will be slower than your normal walking pace—but not always. If you're feeling restless, you may need to walk quickly to discharge energy. If you're feeling sleepy, a brisk pace may wake you up a bit. You might start quickly and then slow down. Or you might start at a snail's pace and then speed up. Remember your mantra: *Go no faster than you can stay connected with feeling.* But also, go no slower. In the middle of a meditation re-treat, your pace may slow down to an almost imperceptible crawl as you savor the exquisite sensation of moving in slow motion. But in the middle of your sped-up daily life, trying to do this might just be irritating.

Begin with the lens of your awareness broad enough to include the whole body. Then, if it feels natural, you can begin to zoom in on the sensation in your legs and feet, particularly the sensation of the soles of your feet contacting the ground. As with any asana, the more sensitively you feel into your lived experience, the more will be revealed to you. Get interested in the feeling of an ankle flexing and extending, a foot lifting and traveling through space. Slow walking can feel like a foot massage—especially if you're lucky enough to be somewhere where you can walk barefoot, such as a sandy beach. Savor the sheer animal pleasure of muscles flexing and joints rolling.

The movement of the feet and legs can reverberate through your whole structure. You're not just walking with your feet—you're walking with your shoulders, neck, spine, and arms.

Especially if you're walking in a beautiful place, your attention may get called away from your body sensations by something in your environment: a lizard doing push-ups on a sun-warmed rock, a blue dragonfly whirring among acacia blossoms, the smell of smoke from a neighbor's fireplace. If so, pause in your walking and open your senses to the smell, sound, or sight. When you've fully absorbed the experience, then continue with your walking practice.

For some people a narrow focus on the feet and legs feels too confining. If that's the case with you, let your awareness lens remain wide. Stay open to the clouds scudding in over the mountains, the distant rumble of traffic, the chirping of the birds, your neighbor's leaf blower, the drumming of rain on your umbrella, the distant tinkle of an ice-cream truck (or the cell phone that sounds like one). Receive the sensory symphony that's playing in, around, and through you.

Remember, there's no one right experience to be having. You're just a human being, walking. That's enough.

PRACTICE 6.33
Walking Meditation II (30–60 minutes)

Compared with the first variation, this variation looks a lot more like taking a walk.

To practice this style of walking meditation, find a place outdoors where you can walk at ease. Don't choose a long hike; pick somewhere you can stroll slowly in the time you have available, attending to the step-by-step experience of walking. If there's natural beauty to refresh your spirits and senses, it's easier to savor your meditation. But you can do this practice anywhere: on city streets, in shopping malls, in airports.

In some ways, this form of walking meditation is more challenging than the first variation—there's more temptation to slip into the delusion that you're trying to get somewhere. So you may want to train up your capacity for walking with presence by practicing the first variation a few times before letting yourself loose in the world. However, for some people, and I count myself among them, it can also feel less forced and more refreshing than a more formal approach. Experiment a little.

After a few minutes of standing meditation, begin your walk. Walk somewhat slower than your normal hiking pace but not so slowly that you'll alarm your neighbors. Let the lens of your awareness be wide and flexible. Can you sense the pressure of your feet on the ground through the skin of your shoes—and at the same time be open to the quarreling of the crows, the warmth of the sun on your neck, the smell of pennyroyal and eucalyptus, the car alarm going off down the block? Call yourself back again and again from your habitual hurry. It's like taking a walk with a child who doesn't care if you ever get to the mailbox. She's happy just poking along, throwing pebbles through gutter grates, marveling equally at dandelions and dog poop.

Imagine that you are caressing the earth with your feet with every step. To heighten your appreciation, Thich Nhat Hanh suggests alternating the words *Yes* and *Thank you* every three steps: *Yes. Yes. Yes. Thank you. Thank you. Thank you.*

If you find that your mind has journeyed light-years into space, try calling yourself back by rotating through your senses. Return to standing meditation for a few breaths, then notice: What are you seeing? What are you hearing? What are you smelling? What are you tasting? What do you feel in your body? Then continue with your walk. Let yourself feel your love for the mysterious, miraculous planet you're walking on.

In Your Asana Practice This Week

In your asana practice this week, spend some extra time on your standing postures. See how it feels to do standing meditation for 5 or 10 minutes before moving into more dynamic postures like Warrior or Triangle. How does that affect your sense of groundedness in your asana practice? How about if you practice the dynamic postures first—does that change your experience in standing meditation? Try doing longer holds than usual of your dynamic standing postures (see practice 2.13 from week 2 on page 69). Especially focus on the sense of energy flowing down through your pelvis, through the legs, and into the earth. Try some one-legged standing balances as well. How is it different to meditate in Tree Pose? Does the added challenge make you more present in your feet and legs? Or do you get caught in striving and self-judgment?

Weave short intervals of walking meditation—just from one end of your mat to the other—into your vinyasa practice. Can you do walking meditation as you go to get your blankets for Shoulder Stand or your blocks and straps?

In Your Daily Life This Week

Once you embrace standing and walking as meditation practices, you'll be astonished at how much more time you have to meditate in your daily life. A simple trip to the bank or the grocery store becomes a chance to rack up those meditation minutes. Instead of cramming in a little extra time on your smartphone, you can meditate while standing in line at the airline check-in counter—or if you leave a little extra time, you can meditate as you walk to your gate, hauling your roller bag behind you. You can meditate standing up on the subway.

Walking Meditation II can be the perfect bridge between a more formal practice and just taking a walk with a bit more mindfulness. Going for a hike with a good friend? Suggest that you do part of it in silence, walking slowly, your senses open. Or take your dog for a meditative stroll.

RESOURCES

Some of my sweetest memories of walking meditation are of walking slowly through golden hills, redwood forests, or fields of sunflowers with hundreds of people on retreats with Thich Nhat Hanh. His book *Walking Meditation* comes with an instructional DVD. For instructions in the vipassana style, there are a number of recorded walking-meditation instructions available at dharmaseed.org. Most of what I know about standing meditation I learned from my partner and qigong teacher, Teja Bell. Check out his website, qigongdharma.com.

WEEK 7

Befriending Your Body

A YOGA TEACHER and psychotherapist recently told me that when he first discovered yoga shortly after graduating from college, he was a hard-core runner and weight lifter struggling with depression, running forty-five miles a week, and "muscle-bound from trying to make myself love myself via weight lifting." Out for a long run one day, Jonathan Reynolds jogged into a yoga studio, picked up a schedule, and jogged straight out again. After his first class, he started practicing yoga every day and never ran or lifted weights again.

But for years he carried over the habit of pushing his body hard in his yoga practice. "All of my running and weight lifting and body-building had been based on self-rejection and body hatred, and I carried that attitude right into my yoga," he told me. "For years I'd hear yoga teachers say things like 'just do your best,' and I'd translate that in my mind as 'try your hardest.' I was forcing myself into asana, with the practice being just another way of constantly telling myself that I wasn't going deep enough, wasn't flexible enough, wasn't good enough."

Like Jonathan, you might have come to yoga drawn by a taste it offers of a different way of being—more joyful, connected, and at ease with yourself and others. But after the initial euphoria wears off, all too quickly the practice can become just another way of beating yourself up. Glance around a yoga class and your worst suspicions are confirmed: *I'm not flexible enough, strong enough, thin enough, or young enough to be here. And my yoga clothes definitely don't cut it!* Yoga puts you face-to-face (or nose to knee, as the case may be) with everything about you that's not working. You can start to feel insecure about body parts you hadn't even known existed previously: *All my life I've felt bad about my butt. But now I feel bad about my psoas as well!*

And let's not even get started on your meditation-impaired mind, scampering around like a chipmunk on a latte. You close your eyes, turn your attention inward, and immediately begin your critique: You're not peaceful enough. You're not kind enough. Your past is riddled with failures. And on top of everything else—you're too judgmental!

Fortunately, the yogic medicine cabinet contains a potent antidote to self-loathing—the systematic cultivation of *metta,* a quality of open-hearted kindness that the Buddha taught as an integral part of meditative awakening. Metta practices can take a lifetime to explore—and there are many wonderful books, talks, and retreats available that delve into them. This week we'll focus on ways to enter the practice of metta through the gate of yoga asana. We'll explore how you can use your asana practice as a place to learn to meet yourself with kindness, how to attune your body to create an inner environment that's supportive of metta meditation, and how to take this embodied feeling of metta and carry it out into your life and relationships.

BUILDING YOUR METTA MUSCLE

Metta is a Pali word that is generally translated as "love" or, more often, "loving-kindness." But one of my favorite translations is "friendliness." Because metta isn't the emotional-train-wreck version of love celebrated in romantic comedies or romance novels. It's not riddled with passion, need, or sentimentality; it's not spiked with possessiveness or the wish to control. Think of the way your dearest friend is always there for you—even when you're being a jerk—and you're getting close to what metta feels like.

And—here's the really good news—metta can be cultivated through formal practice, no matter how challenging your life circumstances. You can grow your ability to greet your tight hamstrings, slipped disks, and sagging skin with as much affection as you do your strong triceps and shining hair. You can learn to accept your frustrations and petty jealousies as well as your luminous moments of generosity and joy. And you can bolster your capacity to wish well-being for everyone from the toll collector on your daily commute to the politicians who most infuriate you.

As a cultivation practice, metta involves not just observing the heart and mind as they are but deliberately inclining them in a particular direction. However, you're not forcing or contriving. Remember how, in weeks 3 and 4, you invited the breath to deepen and lengthen—but only after connecting with and accepting it the way it was? Now you're approaching your heart with the same delicacy and respect. And just as with the breath, it's more about undoing whatever may be blocking your natural capacity for love than it is about manufacturing something new.

In traditional metta meditation, you're instructed to systematically offer love and kindness to yourself and others, focusing your attention through the silent repetition of classic phrases. You begin with yourself: *May I be safe. May I be healthy. May I be joyful. May I be free.* You then extend the same wishes to others: first to a dear friend or benefactor; then to a neutral person, such as a checkout clerk at your local health food store; then to someone you find extremely difficult, such as a challenging in-law. Finally, you extend metta to all beings everywhere, in an expansive blessing that takes in everyone and everything from the mosquito buzzing around your head to whales migrating through Arctic seas.

But metta isn't just an elixir you generate on the meditation cushion. Ultimately, it's meant to infuse the way you meet every inch of your tattered and glorious human life: demolished rain forests and cactus blossoms under a desert moon, your fractured dreams and frayed-around-the-edges triumphs, the people who break your heart and the people who help it mend.

Moving into Metta

In my experience, there are three primary ways that yoga asana practice can help cultivate this quality of openhearted presence:

1. Asana practice can help you *feel* your heart. The increased sensitivity to your inner world that you cultivate through your

asana practice can help you track—without judging—when your heart is contracted or numb and when it's tender and available. You get familiar with the way it opens and closes like a strange and beautiful sea anemone in the shifting currents of your life. And the more intimate you are with this natural pulsation, the more choice you have. It's not that you need to plaster a beaming mask of friendliness over whatever you're really feeling. Rather, you learn to make a kind space for whatever is arising—including, paradoxically, your own closed-heartedness, anger, or disappointment.

2. Asana practice can free your heart. Through conscious movement and breath, you can loosen the conditioned physical and energetic armoring that may block you from accessing your own natural capacity for love. It's not that you have to have open shoulders to have an open heart, and the ability to drop into a back bend from standing is no guarantee that you'll be more compassionate when someone cuts you off on the freeway. But you *can* release habitual neuromuscular patterns that inhibit your natural connection with loving presence.

    If your body is armored in a defensive posture, your muscles and viscera are sending a message to your brain: *Be on guard*. Your nervous system is poised to attack or bolt. When these patterns unwind, your body sends a different message: *It's safe to be vulnerable*. Your nervous system resets for empathy.

    Soften your jaw, and rage may melt into tears. Release your upper back, and the tears may dissolve into gratitude. And as your body releases, kindness may bubble up—not because of a concept that that's how you *should* behave but as an organic expression of who you are.

3. Asana practice can be a garden for growing loving-kindness. Bringing friendliness toward your own body into a yoga practice—rather than striving and competitiveness—can be a potent counterpose to the body-beautiful cult that can subtly (or not so subtly) infiltrate the contemporary yoga scene.

Shining the light of metta into the nooks and crannies of asana practice can illuminate all the ways you might be using your practice to change yourself rather than accept yourself. Not that there's anything wrong with working to become stronger, more flexible, and more balanced. But if what fuels your practice is a feeling of not being good enough, you're doomed. Because no matter what you achieve on the mat, there will always be someone who can do it better. And despite all of your practice, your body is subject to the relentless erosion of time and gravity.

In your yoga practice, you can nurture your ability to be with your physical challenges—that funky hip, that vulnerable neck—not as problems but as parts of you that particularly need your care. When you learn to listen to your aching knee with tenderness, you are more likely to be able to listen to your aching heart or your angry preteen daughter or the guy in your business meeting who won't stop complaining about last quarter's productivity.

And when you stop yanking your body around, you're also less likely to yank your mind around. When you catch your mind wandering in meditation, perhaps you won't whack its little fingers as if you'd caught them in the cookie jar. Instead, you might meet it with kindness and even gratitude: *Hello, planning mind. May you be peaceful. Thank you for your efforts to take care of me.*

Practiced in this way, asana can lay the groundwork for formal seated metta meditation—in which you extend to others the loving-kindness you've been cultivating on the mat—to be not just a mental exercise but an embodied experience. And then you can bring the insights you've generated on the mat and the cushion into your day-to-day interactions.

A HEART BREAKING OPEN ∽ Elaine Conway

Elaine Conway practices yoga in British Columbia.

In 2009, when I had been doing yoga off and on for four or five years, my two children, Fergus and Phoebe, died in a fire at my ex-husband's family cottage on a lake in British Columbia. Fergus was fourteen and Phoebe was eleven.

After my children died, yoga was the only thing I could keep on doing. It was a place I could go and be quiet and not have to talk to people. I was pretty numb, moving very slowly through life. I felt as if I'd been run over by a train and was completely flattened. At my first Easter without my kids, at Easter dinner with my family, everyone was pretending nothing was wrong, and I started to break down. I thought, *I have to go away.* I heard about a twenty-one-day silent vipassana retreat on Hollyhock Island. I couldn't talk to people anymore, I couldn't relate, I couldn't respond—the idea of three weeks in silence sounded like all I could handle.

The retreat started with ten days of metta practice. I had never been on a retreat, and I had never heard of metta before. When people would ask questions about their meditation, I didn't have a clue what anyone was talking about. I was dealing with just one thing, which was the grief. I had this huge lump in my throat and this pain in my heart.

The teachers just kept telling me to take all that pain and meet it with metta, turn it into metta. The metta practice gave me a vehicle for all that pain and also for all that love that was inside all the pain. I couldn't think anymore. I just went inside my body and felt the lump in my throat and the pain in my heart and kept meeting it with love.

By day nine or ten, I started to experience bliss, then rapture. That lasted the rest of the retreat. I was able to hold those polarities of emotion—that incredible joy, along with the deep, deep sorrow and grief. And since the retreat, the practice has allowed me to find that joy and rapture in more and more moments in my everyday life. It happens when I find a deep connection with myself, like when I'm in Savasana or meditating. I've been able to experience so much beauty and so much joy in the rest of my life, even with the sorrow that I still hold.

I've always been a really joyful person. When my kids were alive, we had so much fun together! I've actually almost been fired from jobs for laughing too much. Now, when I have fun and I feel joy, I feel no guilt. I can just really, really feel it.

With my asana practice and teaching now, it's always about metta and compassion. I'm not at all concerned anymore about things like getting into Headstand or Wheel. It's all about compassion. I'll think back on my life with my kids, and inevitably regrets come up. So I need to approach that, too, with compassion. I'm just a much more compassionate person with myself and others.

WEEK 7 PRACTICES

This week, begin every practice period with Setting Your Intention to Be Kind (below). From there, create your asana practice according to the guidelines in Metta in Motion (page 161)—or focus directly on poses to open the heart (page 162). Whatever you do in your asana practice, please be sure you set aside at least 20 to 30 minutes for formal metta practice in your seated meditation posture (page 163).

PRACTICE 7.34
Setting Your Intention to Be Kind (5–10 minutes)

You can do this practice in any stable posture. But I find it particularly powerful to do in a supported heart-opening back bend.

Set a block on its long edge so that the length of the block runs parallel to the end of your mat. Set another block on its end about four inches behind it. (You will need to adjust these distances based on your own body's proportions.) Lie down with your upper back resting on the shorter block, which should be directly behind the heart, supporting the shoulder blades. Support the back of the skull on the taller block. If this is too much of a back bend for you, lower both blocks, so that the lower block is lying on its face and the upper block on its side.

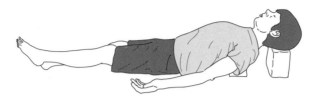

Relax into the support of the props. Although the front of the chest and the sternum are opening, don't strain the heart forward—instead, release it back into the shoulder blades, as if cradled by two hands. Soften the areas that tend to grip—you know them well by now, from your weeks of inner exploration—such as your jaw, the skin on your belly, the muscles around your eyes, your pelvic floor.

Settle your attention in your heart area. Does it feel like a clenched fist? A budding orchid? An ice cube? A hive of buzzing bees? Receive whatever you're feeling with interest and without straining to feel something different. Imagine that your breath is flowing in and out directly through your heart center—bathing it with warmth as you inhale, rinsing out tension and pain as you exhale.

After spending a few minutes connecting with your heart, set your intention to move through your asana and meditation practice today in the spirit of friendship. If it helps, you can focus this intention by silently repeating metta phrases to yourself: *May I be peaceful and joyful. May I meet my body with kindness, just as it is. May my practice be a gift to my body, heart, and mind.* Or you may find it more effective to summon up an image of yourself and invite that image to nestle down into your heart. (If summoning up an image of yourself evokes instant self-criticism—*I can't believe I'm wearing that to appear in a meditation! And look at my hair!*—try visualizing yourself when you were a child instead.)

Now tune in to see if there's any part of your body that needs special attention today: a throbbing knee, an aching back, a gripping in the belly. Again, you might focus your attention with verbal phrases: *May you find ease, aching hip. May you be at peace, clenched jaw.* Set the intention to tend to that part of your body as you practice—not as a problem to be fixed but as something that needs particular tenderness.

When you feel finished, release off the blocks and settle back onto the floor, letting your spine return to its natural curves.

PRACTICE 7.35
Metta in Motion (15–45 minutes)

This practice isn't a prescribed series of postures but an opportunity to amplify and explore metta in any asana sequence you choose—vigorous or restorative, long or short.

After you have completed Setting Your Intention to Be Kind, select the pace, poses, and style of practice that best embody your intention on this particular day. This may vary from one day to the next. If you're coming to your mat after a long day of meetings and e-mails, what feels kindest may be a vigorous sequence of standing poses that wrings tension from your muscles and sends energy coursing through you. If you're exhausted or injured, it may be kindest just to drape yourself over some bolsters and breathe deeply.

Keep checking in throughout your practice, as your needs may change as you enliven your body and become more sensitive to your inner terrain. So don't go on autopilot or work from a script.

If you don't know what to do, try this: Tune in to your body and choose one pose that feels like a gift to yourself. Practice that pose. Then pause, feel inward, and ask: *What might be the next gift I could offer myself?* It's like leaping from one rock to the next across a rushing stream—you don't need to plan the whole journey. Eventually, you'll get to the other side.

If you usually perform a prescribed series of poses, notice where your allegiance to this routine is coming from. Sometimes it's kind to stay with a sequence that you know serves you well. Other times, you may be overriding the pleas of your body out of a contracted sense of duty—loyalty to a practice dictated by "shoulds" and a fear of losing imaginary ground if you don't stick to the form.

Give special attention to the body part that requested it in your opening meditation. Check if you're viewing it as a problem that needs to be fixed or are subtly hoping that if you just give it enough loving-kindness, it will change. What if it never got better? Would you put it out of your heart?

Attend to the way you talk to yourself on the mat. How much of your inner dialogue is oriented toward critiquing what is wrong with your body and your practice—your pooching belly, your wandering mind, the place where your hip freezes during Revolved Triangle? How much does your yoga practice reinforce and refine your ability to criticize yourself rather than strengthen your capacity to wish yourself well?

When you're struggling in a pose, try sending metta to the shoulder or hip or muscle that is squawking the loudest: *May you be happy.* Then let the correct response arrive intuitively: Do you stay in the pose and continue to send metta to that body part? Do you modify the posture? Do you exit the pose altogether? One of the things that's so wonderful about metta in motion is that it's nonprescriptive. It's not dogma but an infinitely creative response to each situation.

Poses to Open the Heart

When practicing metta in motion, you may find it useful to include poses that release the conditioned armoring of the neck, upper back, shoulders, and rib cage—such as back bends, side stretches, and twists. Practice them in a yin or restorative style, with long holds, so you can relax into the openings. And remember to suffuse your practice with the spirit of kindness, letting your poses steep in metta and repeating metta phrases to yourself if that's helpful.

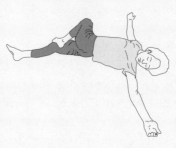

For example, you might drape yourself over a bolster for a supported back bend, then roll onto your side to open your rib cage. A basic reclining twist is delicious for releasing tension in the upper back, right behind the heart. Or you could expand the sides of your rib cage with a Revolved Head to Knee Pose.

When you feel shaky, you'll tend to clench the shoulders and armor the heart. So practice some standing poses, such as Warrior variations, to strengthen your base. Sink roots into the earth and drop your attention into your lower belly and you may find that your heart naturally blooms.

PRACTICE 7.36
Sending Metta to Your Body (10–30 minutes)

This is a variation of Exploring the Whole Body (page 44).

Just as in that practice, set yourself up in a comfortable reclining position and begin moving your attention through your body, inhabiting every hidden room. This time, instead of just sensing your body, actively offer your appreciation to every part of it—your eyes, your ears, your knees, your kidneys, your belly, your big toes. If it helps focus your attention, you can use silent metta phrases: *May you digest with ease, stomach. May you be free of pain, lumbar spine. I'm here to take care of you, hardworking feet.* Or just envelop that body part with the nonverbal attitude of kindness.

Remember to feel the body part as you send your well-wishes, not just visualize it. The more deeply you connect, the more you'll experience the healing benefits. Pay special attention to areas that are injured, ill, neglected, or struggling.

Discover which parts of your body you find easy to cherish, which you judge or reject, and which you skip right over. Sending metta to these different parts of your body can prepare you for sending metta to easy, neutral, and difficult people in your life.

You can do a full body scan in this fashion, or you can spend the entire time focusing on a single area that especially needs your attention. You can also do this practice in a yin or restorative posture.

In Your Seated Meditation Practice This Week

To build on the kindness toward yourself that you've been watering in your asana practice, follow it with a period of seated metta meditation of 20 to 30 minutes.

The following instructions emphasize a sensate approach that naturally grows out of and feeds back into a metta-infused asana practice. Classically, in formal metta meditation you would begin by sending metta to yourself and then widen the circle outward. However, in these instructions I suggest beginning with someone other than yourself, because after a metta-oriented asana practice, it's a natural counterpose to shift your attention outward for a little while.

Begin by tuning in to the feeling in your heart area, as in practice 7.36 (page 163). Breathe a few breaths directly in and out of your heart.

Now think of someone for whom it's very easy for you to feel tenderness—whose imagined presence gives you a feeling of warmth and expansiveness. It doesn't have to be a human; in fact, for many people it's easier if it's not. Try your Labrador retriever, your potted hibiscus, the fawns grazing on your lawn. What's important is that when you think of this creature, you feel an immediate response in your heart, even if it's just a flicker. Visualize this being—let's say it's your dear cat Molly—in vivid detail, as if she were right in front of you. You don't have to strain to see her; just let her appear however clearly or faintly she does. Then invite her right into the center of your heart space. Sense into your natural desire to protect her and wish her well. Notice your natural hope that she be happy, safe, healthy, and free. Notice any physical sensations of softness, warmth, tingling, lightness—and blow on these embers with the breath of your attention so they burn brighter.

If it helps you focus, you can use the classic metta phrases or other ones that work for you: *May you be happy. May you be safe. May you be healthy. May you live at ease.* But if you find the phrases distracting, as many people do, just return to the image and the feeling that goes with it.

Continue to connect with the image and feeling of your beloved cat, or whomever you've chosen, for at least 5 to 10 minutes. (In fact, for your first day, stay with her for the whole meditation, to entrain that friendly feeling into your nervous system.) Keep returning to the feeling, however faint or flickering it is.

When you're ready, let her image dissolve. Now it's time to direct the same feelings of well-wishing toward yourself. Observe what happens at the very suggestion—does your heart, so warm and juicy with affection toward your dear friend curl in on itself like a pill bug? If it's hard for you to summon an image of yourself that you find lovable, think of yourself as a child: recollect that first grade school picture of yourself with the outsized front teeth and the crooked bangs or that baby picture of you banging on your high chair with a sippy cup, strained peas all over your face. Or just open to the formless field of sensations and images and opinions that you call *me* and fold this sense of yourself into your heart like eggs into cake batter.

You can repeat to yourself the metta phrases that work for you: *May I be happy. May I feel loved and accepted just as I am.* Or create your own. But don't get too distracted fiddling around for just the right phrase. You're going for the *feeling* in this embodied approach to practice.

Observe the effects of your metta practice on your body: the subtle and not-so-subtle ways your heart contracts and releases, the tightening or softening of your pelvic floor, the deepening or constriction of your breath.

Some days your heart may feel like a ripe, sweet fruit. On other days it's a hard-shelled nut, and doing metta only seems to irritate you. Try not to use your metta practice as an excuse for beating yourself up about not being more loving. Just as our attempts to focus on the breath illuminate, first of all, how unsteady our minds are, our attempts to contact our innate loving-kindness may immediately illuminate the ways in which we have been conditioned to be less than loving and kind. This does not mean that the practice is not working. On the contrary, it means it's working perfectly.

Send metta to yourself for at least 5 minutes. Don't feel selfish—traditionally, it's common to spend a year sending loving-kindness just to yourself before sending it out to anyone else. We live in a world that's riddled with self-loathing, and ultimately we will treat others as we treat ourselves. So you're doing the world a service by learning to care for yourself.

Metta Blooming

Over time, you can extend your practice to different categories of people, working with them in the same way.

Friends and benefactors. Someone who has been kind to you, mentored you, or offered you support, like your first-grade teacher or your best friend. (It's generally best not to choose your romantic partner for this meditation; unless you're really enlightened, you may have some tiny feelings of attachment mixed in with your metta.)

A neutral person. Someone you know but have no particular feelings toward, such as that woman you pass every morning walking her shih tzu.

A difficult person. The guy who always spreads his mat right next to you in class, a little too close, and then sweats a big puddle. The coworker whose shampoo gives you a headache. (Note: Don't start with the heavy lifting. It's best not to begin with the lover who just left you for someone he or she met on a meditation retreat.)

All beings everywhere. This is often a favorite. (It's much easier to wish all beings well than to well-wish the particular being who just reached their sticky fingers into the bulk granola bin to get another sample.)

As you send metta to friends, acquaintances, and difficult people, remember how you responded to the pleasant, neutral, and difficult sensations in your asana practice. For instance, is there any similarity between the way you responded to your intransigent hip joint and the way you respond to the neighbor who cranks his stereo at midnight?

Many people discover that it's infinitely easier to generate a rush of warmth and tenderness toward a good friend than toward oneself. And one of the blessings of regular metta practice is that it puts you in touch with how many people you love. Metta can connect you, in an instant, to people you care about near and far—from your child asleep in the next room to your high school prom date. Feeling this love can be an immediate, somatic source of nourishment and joy, no matter how much stress you are under.

In Your Life This Week

One of the delights of metta practice is that it's so portable. A moment of metta can transform a routine encounter—with a bus driver, a coworker, even a telemarketer who has interrupted your dinner—into a moment of connection, whether or not the other person is aware of it. (I've heard this referred to as "stealth metta.")

Here are a few suggestions for portable metta practice (feel free to create your own):

E-mail metta. Before you send an e-mail, take a moment to send metta to the recipient: *May you be happy. May you be free.* Then hit Send. (Or, as the case may be, reconsider whether you want to send that particular message at all.)

Falling-asleep metta. As you lie in bed, instead of retraveling the day's peaks and swamps in your mind, send metta to yourself and the people you love. (I've found metta particularly helpful when struggling with insomnia.)

Headline metta. When you read a news story or watch a television report, send metta to all the people involved. See what it's like to send it with impartiality to all candidates—for instance, when following an election—or to both perpetrator and victim when the news is of a crime. Pay particular attention to the sensations in your body as you do that.

Traffic metta. Use every stoplight as an opportunity to send metta to the people in the cars in front of or behind you. The same for traffic jams and stalled cars. Some jerk cut you off on the freeway? Send the driver a metta blast instead of a muttered curse.

Cooking metta. Imagine the faces of the friends and family who will eat a dish you are preparing and send them love as you chop the onions, crush the garlic, grate the cheese. Then send them a little more as you scrape their plate scraps into the compost, wash the thumbprints off their glasses.

RESOURCES

You can't go wrong with Sharon Salzberg's classic book *Lovingkindness: The Revolutionary Art of Happiness* or Jack Kornfield's *The Art of Forgiveness, Lovingkindness, and Peace.* Loving-kindness meditations guided by both Sharon and Jack are available through Sounds True. Also check out *May I Be Happy,* a memoir about self-love and yoga by OM yoga founder Cyndi Lee.

I Love It! I Hate It!
I'm Bored to Death!

WHEN SKYE WAS TWO years old, I gave him his first Popsicle on a hot July day. He was snuggling in my lap as we rocked in the bench swing next to the lavender bushes in our backyard. With his first few licks of icy orange, his face lit up: "This is so yummy!" He took another slurp and proclaimed cheerfully, "And when this Popsicle is all gone, I'll have *another* one!"

Foolishly, I hastened to set him straight: "Oh, no, sweetie, one will be plenty. Too much sugar's not good for you."

He pulled the Popsicle out of his mouth and began to howl. "I want *another* one!"

I tried to point out that he actually already had a Popsicle he hadn't eaten yet. But ignoring the melting one in his hand, he went on wailing because he couldn't have seconds.

How many times have you let a delectable experience melt away, unable to enjoy it fully because you know it's going to end and you won't get more? As you already know from paying attention to the territory of your body and mind, you live in a never-ending river of sensory experiences—temple bells and jackhammers, honeysuckle and rotting garbage, chocolate and sour milk, velvet and nettles. Some of them you like. Some you don't like. Some you don't care about one way or another. And they are always changing. You're sunbathing on a beach and the wind starts blowing sand in your face. You're laid off your job and finally have time to write a screenplay.

So how do you live with ease in the middle of such instability? What will bring a reliable sense of contentment?

The liberating insight offered by the Buddha is that happiness is not determined by what's going on at any given moment. It's how we relate to these changing circumstances that determines the quality of our life.

According to the Buddha's map of our inner terrain, whenever a physical or mental phenomenon arises in our awareness, we experience it as colored by a feeling tone, or *vedana,* of pleasant, unpleasant, or neutral. Left unnoticed, each of these primary feeling tones can trigger a whole chain reaction of emotions and behaviors—some of them life enhancing, others . . . well, less so. The key for our mindfulness practice is to become more and more aware of these simple feeling tones and our reactions to them before they set off full-blown emotional dramas. Then we have more choice in how we respond moment to moment to the flow of our lives. This conscious investigation is the territory of what the Buddha called the second foundation of mindfulness.

When I first heard mindfulness of feeling tones explained, I thought it sounded incredibly dry and robotic. Was I supposed to pare down my entire vibrant emotional palette to these three primary colors? Even more off-putting: was there something *wrong* with enjoying pleasant things and steering clear of unpleasant ones? I wanted to get in touch with the jungle drums of Eros, the wailing violins of grief. I didn't want to reduce my life to a vedana-powered binary code.

But when I entered into it as a living practice, I began to realize its power. Mindfulness of feeling tones isn't a dampening down of life but an opening to its moment-to-moment flickering. We're not trying to get rid of these primary feeling tones or even our responses to them; we're receiving them with heightened sensitivity. That way we can savor enjoyable moments—the smell of coffee and banana muffins, the sun glinting off puddles as we dash toward a bus, our grandmother's smile—without compulsively chasing after them or trying to preserve them in formaldehyde. We can choose to initiate that painful but necessary conversation with the friend who let us down. We can stop running away from our own brokenheartedness or someone else's.

This week we will be using our asana and meditation practice to explore our relationship with these primary feeling tones and to train ourselves to relate to them in a skillful way. We'll use our asana practice as a laboratory in which we consciously create and study pleasant, unpleasant, and neutral experiences—and our own reactions to them—to deepen our understanding of how to live with wisdom and ease.

PLEASANT: "THIS IS GREAT! GIMME MORE!"

Let's face it—we hatha yogis and yoginis come to yoga largely because it feels good. We love wringing out tension from tight muscles and sweating out stress from every pore. Some of us love the burn of a sweaty vinyasa; others melt to the surrender of lying on our backs with our legs up the wall and a lavender-scented pillow over our eyes. But whether our practice of choice is a yin-style forward bend or a series of handstand drop backs, we tend to be pleasure junkies—if it didn't feel so good, we probably wouldn't keep coming back.

And yet if we're not conscious, we can race right by these delicious sensations without fully savoring them—straining toward the next pose and the next and the next, as if the point of our practice were to score as many pleasant moments as possible.

This cascade of grasping is a typical response to a pleasant experience. *This is good! How can I keep it from stopping? How can I get more and keep it forever?* Left unexamined, this reflexive clutching can poison a moment's pleasure—a kiss, a walk in a meadow, a cup of steaming cider—with anxiety and dissatisfaction. And it can trigger a chain reaction of plotting and manipulation as you chase the unattainable goal of surrounding yourself entirely with what's pleasurable, as if your life could be an endless vinyasa consisting only of your favorite poses, all performed flawlessly to the applause of an adoring crowd.

Mindfulness practice—and in particular, the kind of embodied mindfulness that we are cultivating in this program—helps you avoid this painful trap in several ways. First of all, it helps you recognize and appreciate pleasant sensations as they happen.

You can soak in joy by becoming attentive to the bare experience of pleasure itself—knowing that an experience is delightful as it is happening. By becoming aware of the pleasant nature of sensations as they blossom, you turn up the volume on the background level of sweetness in your life.

Contemporary neuroscience reveals, as the psychologist and mindfulness teacher Rick Hanson explains in his excellent book *Buddha's Brain,* that the human brain is "like Velcro for negative experiences, Teflon for positive ones." It has evolved to scan the environment for threats and learn quickly from negative experiences. When something unpleasant occurs, the record of this event immediately gets etched into your neural circuits, where it becomes part of your "implicit memory"—the largely unconscious brain mapping that informs your ongoing sense of happiness or unhappiness. Pleasant experiences, on the other hand, evaporate from your brain like mist in the sun if they are not consciously opened to. Left unnoticed, they are not transferred from short-term to long-term storage.

But here's some good news: If you let yourself marinate in these pleasant experiences consciously for at least thirty to forty seconds, they write themselves into your brain and nervous system. They become part of a background hum of your circuitry that steadily feeds your ongoing sense of well-being.

You can use this principle to enhance your pleasure in your asana practice. As you move into a pose that feels good, really let yourself *know* that it feels good. Take a few breaths to soak in the hum in your spine as you arc into a back bend, the release of your sacrum as you pour forward over your legs. Slow your flow down enough to let your nervous system fully register its delight. Open to the deep sense of well-being that comes from caring well for your precious human body.

Shallow Pleasures

However, mindfulness is not just about turning up the volume on pleasure. If your practice stops there, you risk being trapped in a shallow, bliss-bunny understanding of yoga. What happens to your practice when you're sick or injured? What happens when you have to walk barefoot through the shattered glass of a broken heart? To be meaningful, savoring pleasant moments must be accompanied by an increased capacity to tolerate—and even embrace—the truth that reveals itself as soon as you pay attention: that even as you enjoy these pleasant feelings, they are melting away.

Triangle Pose morphs into Warrior, Warrior dissolves into a back bend, Back Bend dissolves into Savasana, and before you know it you have rolled up your mat and are back in freeway traffic. The lover kissing you will grow old and die. The child giggling in your lap will grow into the teenager who finds you embarrassing.

This realization knocks the legs out from under a yoga practice fixated on hedonism. In a culture oriented toward instant gratification, happiness looks like an ad I recently saw in a catalogue: a couple relaxing in an outdoor heated swimming pool, watching a romantic comedy on a giant weatherproof video screen, with a remote-controlled cooler on wheels trundling them cold beers at the touch of a button. In that universe, the ultimate goal of your practice is an exquisitely appointed home yoga studio where you strut through your most flattering asanas, dressed in designer yoga wear, in a body that's eternally flexible, healthy, strong, and twenty-three years old.

But there's a desperate uneasiness in this vision, because we intuitively sense that it's built on a foundation of Jenga blocks. Inevitably, life—in the form of a stage 4 cancer, a ruptured disk, the death of a dear friend—will come along and yank one block out, and the whole precarious edifice will come crashing down.

A mindful yoga practice opens the door to a joy that's deeper than a stream of pleasant moments. It takes us on a tour through poses we love, poses we hate, poses we're indifferent to. And the real yoga comes when we learn to receive the lessons each has to teach us, not gloating when we do well or flinching away when it's difficult. We learn to savor our pleasures without blindly chasing them or strangling the ones we already have in a death grip of attachment.

Knowing on a cellular level that things are constantly changing, we start to see through our mind's glib assumptions about what brings happiness. We learn to discriminate between pleasures that lead to joy and health for ourselves and others and those that lead to addiction and suffering. I love chocolate—but if I eat it at night, I can't sleep. So the pleasant sensation of a big slice of chocolate cake after dinner contains the seeds of the unpleasant sensation of tossing and turning late into the night, unable to find a lump-free spot on my pillow, worrying about crashing hard drives, melting glaciers, and missed deadlines.

So I usually choose to pass on the chocolate cake. This decision isn't about the virtuous non–cake eater inside me arresting the criminal cake eater and handcuffing her. It's a spontaneous sensing of what will really bring me long-term well-being. And sometimes I choose to have a bite or two of chocolate cake anyway—enough to sweeten the moment without poisoning the whole night. I let myself savor each mouthful. *Mmmmm. Pleasant.*

UNPLEASANT: "I HATE THIS! MAKE IT STOP!"

Years ago a student on a yoga and meditation retreat told me that she had a strong aversion to hip openers: the asanas like Pigeon Pose that stretch those tight bands of muscle around the outsides of the hips. Holding Pigeon for more than a few minutes, Suzanne wouldn't just get uncomfortable—she'd get furious. She'd come on this yoga and meditation retreat hoping to find some inner peace. But instead, it seemed that every five minutes—there came another hip opener! She'd spent most of the afternoon's yin yoga session simmering with rage—first toward her tight hips, then toward the retreat teachers and the yogis on the mats around her, and ultimately toward the entire twenty-five-hundred-year lineage of male, patriarchal, hip-hostile Buddhist meditation practice.

You may have a pose or two that makes you feel like that—most of us do. Generally, they're the ones that don't come easily, that target the places in your body where you're tight or weak. You never seem to get around to them in your home practice, and when you see them approaching in a yoga class, you want to hide in the bathroom.

It's natural, and sometimes intelligent, to want to bolt from unpleasant experiences. But if you're not conscious of this natural impulse, it can rule your life. You might zone out on sugar or online videos rather than face boredom, depression, or despair. You might have an affair rather than open up the painful conversation about what's not working in your relationship. You might turn away from the news about global environmental collapse because it's simply too hard to bear.

But no matter how you bolt the doors, life will climb in your window with its armfuls of sorrow. Even if you've miraculously kept it out for a lifetime, loss will catch up with you at the finish line, delivering on the promise of impermanence that has lurked around the edges of your most spectacular accomplishments.

Mindfulness invites a different choice—to open to unpleasant experiences as they arise and investigate their nature. This doesn't mean that you seek out pain for its own sake or intentionally stay in situations that cause harm to you or other people. But it means that moving away from discomfort, or staying and working within it, becomes a choice, not a reflex.

Just as with mindfulness of pleasant sensations, mindfulness of unpleasant sensations begins with a simple acknowledgment of what's true. Preparing your breakfast, you open what looks like a tub of yogurt and are greeted with the festering smell of two-week-old leftover Thai food. You find out that the ex who broke your heart has just gotten married on a Maui beach. Your first impulse may be to spin out into a story: *Why doesn't your roommate/significant other ever throw out his leftovers? And your ex had insisted that it wasn't about you, she just didn't believe in the institution of marriage! What is wrong with these people?* But instead, you pause. You sense your stomach churning as you smell rotting pad thai. You feel your breath tighten as you see photos online of the happy couple at their honeymoon luau. And you notice: *Ah. This is unpleasant.*

Often, simply acknowledging to yourself that an experience is unpleasant opens up space around it. It gives the moment room to breathe, so you can realize that maybe you don't need to ask your roommate to move out. Maybe you don't need to post embarrassing pictures of your ex online to retaliate. You can just be with the unpleasant sensations as they roll through you. Then you can choose—from a place of balance—how you want to respond.

Opening the arms of your awareness to include what is uncomfortable or painful—rather than trying to run from it or push it away—can be a tremendous relief. You can welcome all of yourself home—including the parts that you may have exiled from your awareness as too painful, too embarrassing, too damaged.

As her meditation retreat progressed, Suzanne discovered that her asana practice could be a powerful forum for cultivating this capacity to just be with unpleasant sensations. Together we ascertained that she wasn't injuring her body in the hip-opening poses. She was just feeling the physical discomfort of tight muscles stretching and the emotions they released as they unwound. So I encouraged her to use the sensitivity she'd been cultivating on the meditation retreat to investigate the sensations in her hips, beginning with short holds—just a minute or so on each side—to move gently into the tissues without overwhelming her nervous system.

As she felt the burning in her outer hips, she learned to soften around it. She didn't need to create a story, she realized; she could just name the sensation as unpleasant and then make the choice to rest with it a little longer. When she didn't harden around the feelings or believe the stories her mind was spinning, the discomfort just wasn't that big a deal. As the retreat progressed, her hip openers became a place for her to practice working with a resistance to uncomfortable experiences that impeded other areas of her life as well.

Choosing Discomfort

This ability to choose to be with what's unpleasant—while discerning between what's merely unpleasant and what's injurious—opens up a tremendous freedom, especially as you work with more complex emotions. You can choose to speak uncomfortable truths, knowing that you can tolerate the feelings of embarrassment or discomfort that may arise when other people get angry. You develop the capacity to be with intense emotions—your own and other people's—without getting overwhelmed.

This doesn't mean that you seek out or perpetuate damaging situations. In fact, sometimes the realization that something is unpleasant becomes your cue to remove yourself: *This pose is sending sharp pains through my knee, and that's probably injurious. I'm going to back off.* Or, *Every time I go out for coffee with this person, I end up feeling like a total loser. Maybe I won't hang out with her anymore.*

But being able to tolerate strong, unpleasant sensations in the body—whether physical or emotional—gives you the freedom to make wise choices, even if doing so entails some discomfort. It's the power to go for a run around a lake on a winter day rather than eat chips in front of the TV. It's the power to stand for hours in a cold rain protesting an unjust war.

To get to that deeper power of yoga, you have to be willing to go into territory that's uncomfortable. You have to learn to sit with the aching muscle, the stubborn joint, and discern between the discomfort that leads to opening and healing and the discomfort that causes injury. And you have to come to terms with the fact that sometimes the injury won't heal and the pain won't go away.

Along the way, you may realize that some of your assumptions about what is unpleasant are not entirely accurate. As you hold an asana you've been resisting, you may discover that what you have been reflexively labeling as "pain" and flinching away from is, in fact—when you look more closely—a pulsing vibration that is at times intensely pleasurable. Just as some pleasant sensations contain the seeds of suffering, some unpleasant ones contain the seeds of delight. The burn in your quads as you hike up a mountain trail is entwined with the joy of being outdoors. The uncomfortable throb in your shoulders as you hold a long Downward Dog is inseparable from the pleasure you feel in growing stronger.

Recently I ran into Suzanne in the produce aisle of the market, picking out avocados. She told me that these days, hip openers are her favorite pose.

NEUTRAL: "I'M BORED!"

When my niece Montana was six years old, my sister and her husband took her on a long-anticipated family sabbatical in Europe. They had planned the journey for months, and her excitement had built to a fever pitch. But when she walked out the doors of the airport in Rome, she took one look around at the busy streets and burst into tears. "This isn't *Europe*," she sobbed. "This is just a *place*!"

We'd like our life to be a journey from one peak experience to the next—an unending vinyasa of beautiful poses. But in fact, large stretches are generally uneventful. And even the experiences we think of as most exciting—like a trip to Europe—are largely composed of mundane details. Many of life's most dramatic experiences—both pleasant and unpleasant—actually consist primarily of ordinary moments. Traveling through India, I was amazed how much of my spiritual pilgrimage was spent standing in line at a post office, rinsing out dirty socks and underwear in ashram sinks and hanging them to dry on a laundry line stretched between a door handle and a windowsill. On your honeymoon in Maui, you'll still have to blow your nose and wash your hair.

These are what Buddhist psychology terms the neutral moments—the unassuming sensations that arrive unheralded by the flutes of pleasure or the trumpets of pain. Instead of dancing the rumba with a lampshade on their head, neutral experiences sit quietly in their librarian glasses on the edge of the party, where your attention slides right over them.

In your yoga practice, neutral moments aren't the blissful rushes in your spine or the throbbing burn in your quads. They're the pressure of your sitting bones against the floor, the turning of your shoulder in its socket, the beating of your heart, the steady movement of your breath in and out. In your life, they're the packing pellets between the "valuable" events—making your bed, brushing your teeth, dropping a sock in your laundry basket, sitting in the car while the long miles of prairie highway unfurl behind you.

We don't tend to chase after neutral feelings, and we don't run away from them. In fact, most of the time we don't pay much attention to them at all. But here's the thing—these neutral moments actually make up a huge proportion of our experience. So if we miss them, we miss a lot of our life.

Savoring the Mundane

Your asana practice is a great place to train yourself to notice these subtle experiences. For example, you can learn to pay attention to the transitions between poses as well as the poses themselves. What do you feel as you travel in and out of Triangle Pose? What sensations do you notice as you make your way from standing down to the ground?

As you hold a pose, you can look beyond the obvious primary sensations of stretch, tingle, and burn to the background feeling of your feet in contact with the mat, the movement of breath in your pelvic floor, the sensation in the palm of a hand as it moves through space.

And as you do this, you may discover something remarkable: that when you pay attention to neutral sensations, they often alchemically transform into pleasant ones. The seemingly neutral backdrop of your ordinary experience can become a source of delight, simply through the power of your mindful presence.

As Zen master Thich Nhat Hanh points out in his book *Peace Is Every Step*, "When we have a toothache, we know that not having a toothache is a wonderful thing. But when we do not have a toothache, we are still not happy. A non-toothache is very pleasant." Paying attention to your body, you can open to a wellspring of gratitude for the injuries you don't have. You can become grateful for having eyes that can see, ears that can hear, skin that can feel the cool breeze off the ocean or the pressure of a child's hand in yours. Opening to the neutral experiences in life can actually alter the neural substrate of your experience, laying down a background sense of contentment that emanates from your implicit memory.

In your asana practice, you can nourish appreciation for the neutral moments by sending gratitude to your body—particularly the parts that aren't currently screaming for your attention. You can appreciate your feet for carrying you to and through your practice. You can appreciate your fingers as they deftly wrap around your big toe. You can appreciate all the physical systems—heart, lungs, brain, lymph—that are working in seamless, largely invisible synchrony to make your life possible.

One of the great gifts of the practice of noticing pleasant, unpleasant, and neutral is that we become aware that our experience, which seems so solid, is actually an ever-flowing river of sensations, each drop with its own feeling tone. These moments constantly eddy and swirl, creating a multidimensional and nuanced experience. You are spending a romantic weekend in a bed-and-breakfast—and your soul mate wakes up next to you with rancid morning breath. You are sitting in a lawyer's office signing your divorce papers, and the smell of the honeysuckle through the window is sweet.

As you cultivate your ability to swim in that river, you find that your yoga practice is bringing you to a steadier, truer kind of happiness than you could ever arrive at by simply chasing after one blissful pose after another.

FINDING FREEDOM BEHIND BARS   〰   Leslie Booker

Leslie Booker teaches yoga and meditation to incarcerated youth in New York City.

In New York City, kids are locked up as young as seven. The youngest kid I've worked with was age ten. A lot of these kids were looking at life sentences. When you're working with a fourteen-year-old who is going to spend the rest of his life in jail—that's intense.

People sometimes think that teaching yoga and meditation to kids is about teaching them to be really great yogis, but it's not about that at all. It's about teaching them to have more awareness and choice in their lives so they have more control over their emotions and can make better choices.

Learning to identify pleasant, unpleasant, and neutral experiences was such a breakthrough for me, both in my own practice and in working with the kids. A lot of these kids have had so much trauma, and a lot of them are dealing with drugs and alcohol addiction on top of everything else. They are so quick to jump out of their bodies, to jump out of what's uncomfortable. That's a lot of what happens with trauma—we don't want to feel our pain, so we escape with drugs or high-risk behavior or promiscuous behavior.

Sometimes uncomfortable feelings come up in our yoga sessions. We have a contract with each other that no matter what happens, we're not allowed to leave the circle.

I have the kids learn how to check in with themselves. If they're in the middle of a hip opener and it's unpleasant, can they just sit with it a few breaths instead of saying "I'm out of here"? I give them permission to say "This sucks, I hate this" and still sit with the feeling. That way they can become friends with their feelings in their own bodies.

A lot of these kids are in prison because they reacted too fast. Someone says something to them, they get mad, suddenly they're beating someone up, and then their hands are in handcuffs—*whoa, how did that happen?* Yoga helps them learn to slow down so they can feel what triggers in their body. I'll ask someone, "What happened right before you hit that person?"

"Oh, I got that bad feeling in my gut."

"What would happen if you just felt that bad feeling instead of hitting him?"

They start to see they have some choices. Someone will come to me and say, "Booker, this kid was talking shit to me, and three weeks ago I would have hauled off and hit him. But I thought about what you said and I didn't hit him." Or "This girl was mouthing off and I realized I was really mad. So instead of yelling back I just walked away and came back when I was calm."

I tell kids, "They can't imprison your mind." I'm not teaching kids to escape their reality but to get clear and present with what their reality is and see where they have choices in this situation. If a kid is going to be locked up in solitary confinement for days, I tell the kid, "You have your body, you have your breath, you have your mind. What can you do with this?"

WEEK 8 PRACTICES

This week's practices are not so much about what you are *doing* as what you are *paying attention to*. Following are three different approaches to an asana practice focusing on mindfulness of feeling tones, each one about 30 to 60 minutes: Noticing Feeling Tones in Long Holds (page 182), A Few of Your Favorite Things (page 183), and Hard Times (page 184). Each day select one of these practices to focus on. Follow your asana practice with at least 20 to 30 minutes of seated meditation that includes mindfulness of pleasant, unpleasant, and neutral sensations (page 184).

PRACTICE 8.37
Noticing Feeling Tones in Long Holds (30–60 minutes)

One of the best ways to study your reactions to pleasant, unpleasant, and neutral sensations is to hold your yoga postures longer than usual. Most of us have an unconscious inner timer that regulates how long we hold a posture before we get restless and move on. Hold past your comfort zone and interesting feelings bubble up.

Set a timer to chime every 5 minutes. (If you already know you are comfortable in that rhythm, set it for longer. Seven minutes? Nine? Notice when the number sets off a frisson of anxiety—*That might hurt! That sounds really boring!*—and set it there.) Then move through a series of long-held yoga poses, including both poses that come easily and ones that are more challenging.

Yin poses are great for this kind of practice because they can be held for long periods without injury while creating strong sensations. But it's also interesting to experiment with more active poses, such as Downward Dog or Trikonasana, that can be held without risking injury to vulnerable areas such as the spine or knees.

Settle into each pose with a spacious, open attention. After attending to the basic details of alignment that create safety and ease, rest your attention in the sensations of breath and body. Check into where your attention naturally gravitates: The movement of the breath? Refining the details of your alignment? The strong sensations the pose creates in a particular area?

As you hold the pose, the sensations will probably start to intensify. Take these strong sensations as the focal point of your attention. Just as you did in week 2, get interested in the precise details of your experience: tingling, burning, throbbing, pulsing. And also notice: Do you experience these feelings as pleasant? Unpleasant? Or neither? Do you find yourself wanting to get away from them? Or to go deeper into them? Don't spend a lot of time analyzing; if a feeling tone doesn't immediately announce itself, just let the sensation continue to blossom.

Notice any tendency to want to amplify or prolong the pleasant sensations. There's no need to judge this impulse—it's a normal human response. Instead, get curious: Where in your body do you feel this grasping impulse? Is the feeling of grasping itself pleasant or unpleasant? Does it add to or detract from your ability to receive the pleasure? See if you can soften the grasping wherever it lives in your body (a subtle tightness in the back of the skull, a tongue pressed hard against the roof of your mouth) while still fully enjoying the pleasure.

Also notice any impulse to avoid the unpleasant sensations—either by contracting away from them or pushing them away from you. Again, this is an instinctive biological response—so don't judge or try to get rid of it. Just notice: Where does aversion live in your body? Is the feeling of contraction or pushing away pleasant or unpleasant? What happens if you soften into and around the aversion itself? Try just naming the experience: *My hip is burning and tingling. It is unpleasant.* How does it feel to include what's unpleasant in the embrace of your awareness?

If there doesn't seem to be much going on, do you check out? Instead, inquire into this "neutral" experience. What subtle feelings are emerging? Can you get really interested in what it feels like to be bored?

As the minutes tick by, notice whether you're waiting impatiently for the timer to chime. Then notice your feelings when it does. Is there relief as you come out of the pose? Disappointment?

PRACTICE 8.38
A Few of Your Favorite Things (30–60 minutes)

For this practice, create a yoga sequence consisting entirely of your very favorite postures, pranayamas, and flows—a whole vinyasa of raindrops on roses and whiskers on kittens. You can plan it in advance or just let it emerge spontaneously from one pose to the next—Mmm, that felt great; what do I want to do next?

Let this be an exercise in savoring delight. As you begin your yoga sequence, consciously register the pleasure you feel in every gesture. Let it radiate from the core of the stretch out through your whole body and beyond. Soak fully in each experience before moving on.

Sometimes our minds skitter away from pleasure even more than they do from pain, as if it threatens our whole sense of identity simply to feel good. Are you spacing out and missing moments of joy? Do you feel that you're cheating by not doing something more challenging?

Investigate any gap between what you think is pleasant and what actually gives you satisfaction. Do your favorite poses contain moments of discomfort? Do you enjoy *doing* your practice as much as *having done* it?

Just as in practice 8.37, notice whether your pleasure in your practice is accompanied by a feeling of grasping—a contraction around the pleasure in an attempt to hold on to it. Does the grasping enhance your pleasure? Or impede it?

PRACTICE 8.39
Hard Times (30–60 minutes)

You knew this was coming. . . . Now create a practice composed primarily of your least favorite poses—the ones you're not good at or that set your teeth on edge. Don't choose risky asanas that you're not physically prepared for—just ones that give you a sinking feeling inside when your teacher suggests them.

As you move into the sequences of poses you have created, notice what makes them unpleasant: A strong physical sensation? The frustration of not being able to do them "right"? An unsettling emotion they squeeze out of your tissues? What does it feel like to just name this feeling as "unpleasant" and continue with the posture? Are there moments of pleasure buried inside your exploration of a posture you think you don't like?

As you rest in Savasana at the end of your practice, how does your body feel? How about your heart? How about your mind?

In Your Seated Meditation This Week

Be sure to take at least 20 to 30 minutes each day for your seated meditation this week—long enough for some challenges to emerge. At the beginning of your practice, take a couple of minutes to acknowledge any ease, openness, or other positive sensations that may already be present—as well as tuning in to see where you might be feeling pain or discomfort. Then settle your focus on your body and breath.

When you find that you have been swept away by a tidal wave of thoughts, take a moment to notice, before returning to your anchor, not just what has swept you away but what its feeling tone is. Were you lost in pleasant fantasies? Apocalyptic worries? Or were you just spacing out? Don't think about this too much. Just notice if a feeling tone announces itself. Give it an inner bow of acknowledgment: *Greetings, pleasant daydream. Greetings, painful knot in the middle of my upper back.* Taste its pleasant or unpleasant quality. Then ease your attention back to your anchor.

In Your Daily Life This Week

As you flow through the vinyasa of your life, continue to open to the feeling tone of your experience. Pay particular attention to the surprising nuances. You may think of washing dishes as unpleasant, but do your hands feel good as you plunge them into the warm, soapy water? You may enjoy travel, but is it pleasant to sit on an airplane for seven hours? And what about those neutral periods where you just space out? When you pay attention there, what blossoms?

RESOURCES

Rick Hanson's books *Buddha's Brain* and *Hardwiring Happiness* are readable resources for understanding the neuropsychology of how our brains are wired to respond to pleasant, unpleasant, and neutral sensations. Thich Nhat Hanh's *Present Moment, Wonderful Moment* offers poetic and practical guidance for transforming neutral experiences into pleasant ones.

Coming Home to Your Heart

Yogis on meditation retreats often report unusually vivid dreams—a dialing up of the unconscious as the conscious mind gets quieter, just as the stars blaze brighter in the night sky when you're camping miles from the city lights.

A few years ago I led a small women's retreat in a cloistered meditation room on the second floor of a retreat center. Meanwhile, downstairs in the main temple, sixty-five psychotherapists were attending a different silent retreat. On the third night—as the pressure cooker of intensive practice was starting to steam—I dreamed that all of the psychotherapists had brought their craziest clients along with them. The retreat center had transformed into a B-movie version of a lunatic asylum—yogis were wandering around in various stages of mental disintegration, wailing and tearing their hair. One therapist looked just like Miss Trunchbull, the evil school principal in the children's movie *Matilda* who was always threatening to lock misbehaving kids in a dark closet bristling with metal spikes. Brandishing a gag at one of her clients, Miss Trunchbull was hissing, "If you don't settle down, you *know* I'm going to have to restrain you!"

That's exactly how meditation practice sometimes feels. When we come to our practice, we all bring our craziest clients with us—the raging, grieving, wild aspects of our psyches. And we also get in touch with the inner Miss Trunchbull, who just wants the crazies to shut up, even if it means gagging them.

Encountering these characters can be a shock. You sit down on your cushion expecting meditation to be blissful, or at least manageable. After all, how hard can it be just to sit and be present with yourself for a half hour, an hour, a day, or a week? And then the inner voices start to rant. Decades ago, I read a book that cheerfully proclaimed, "Meditation is like eating a delicious, cool ice-cream cone on a hot summer day." "No," I thought, setting the book down. "Meditation is like being locked in a dark closet with a lunatic with a megaphone."

This lunatic may be sobbing, shrieking, laughing, or dancing. She may be berating you for all the idiotic things you've done or the brilliant things you haven't. He may be recounting conversations you had with your high school girlfriend twenty years ago or would like to have with your boss next week. She is passionate, regretful, ecstatic, jealous, truculent—and totally, *totally* out of your control.

Fortunately, you don't have to brandish a gag. Mindfulness is not about converting your inner nuthouse into a cloister of silent, celibate monks and nuns reciting their rosaries. It's about getting to know who's in there and what they might have to tell you.

For the next few weeks, we'll be focusing on using our yoga practice to support a wise relationship with the denizens of this inner world. This is the territory of what Buddhist psychology calls the third foundation of mindfulness, commonly translated as "mindfulness of the mind."

Remember that in the language of the Buddha and the ancient yogis, *heart* and *mind* were the same word. Most modern practitioners, however, experience them as two separate though tightly knit phenomena: the emotions as the raw contents of our heart and the thoughts as the verbal narrative in our head that both triggers and tries to explain them. So we'll focus our investigations this week on emotional content before turning our attention to the nature of the storytelling mind.

Remember, though, that our emotions can power the projector in the movie theater of our heads. The stories we tell ourselves can ignite a firestorm in the dry brush of our hearts. So in exploring our emotions, we're inevitably examining the nature of our thoughts as well. And in investigating with thoughts, we wind our way back to the emotions that fuel them.

GETTING TO KNOW THE EMOTIONAL BODY

In your yoga over the past several weeks, you've been consciously moving into the dark, neglected corners of your body—loosening what's stuck, feeling what's numb, melting frozen rivers. And when you do this, you're inevitably doing the same thing with your emotional body. You might roll out of Shoulder Stand and burst into tears. You might release from a back bend into a gale of giggles.

Your life experiences are trapped in clenched jaws and diaphragms. They are inscribed in your neural networks, woven into your myofascial webs. And so when you open your body, out dance ghosts and demons, blissful and wrathful *dakinis*, jesters and fools.

In yogic cosmology, thoughts and emotions inhabit the realm of the manomayakosha, or mental body—which overlaps and permeates both the physical body (annamayakosha) and the breath and energy body (pranamayakosha). (For a refresher on the koshas, see The Body-Mind Matrix, on page 31.) Body, breath, heart, and mind are constantly in communication.

You don't have to buy into yogic cosmology to see this interplay at work. As you check your e-mail, sense your clenched neck: *I'm terrified I won't get everything done on my list, and people will realize that I'm not good enough!* Reaching for the cheese platter at the crowded party, feel the tight jaw beneath your plastered-on smile: *My pants are too tight, the music is too loud, and this person's view on climate change is really pissing me off.*

In the song of your body, the voices of past and present twine together: the smack of Sister Mary Monica's ruler on your five-year-old palm, the whiplash crack of your neck as your prom-night car spun out of control on the icy bridge, the grief handed down the generations from a great-great-grandfather in chains.

The second line of Patanjali's Yoga Sutra—often quoted in yoga classes—is *"Yoga citta vritti nirodha,"* which is generally translated as some variation on "Yoga is the stilling of the fluctuations of the mind." This can create a misperception among yogis that to do yoga and meditate properly, we need to silence our emotions and thoughts.

But mindfulness of the emotions isn't about scrubbing them away with spiritual Ajax as if they're a nasty stain on the pristine bathtub of our consciousness. Emotions—even the grubby, painful, or embarrassing ones—are a vital part of the ecosystem of our psyche, as natural and essential as swallows darting in the oak branches or worms tunneling through the banana peels in the compost bin. Mindfulness is about opening to a wise and connected relationship with them while also sensing that we are larger than they are. I like the yoga teacher Richard Miller's translation of *Yoga citta vritti nirodha*: "Yoga is when we abide in and as our True Nature—Stillness—that is without movement, whether the mind, which is the movement of thought, is in movement or not."

In his instructions on the third foundation of mindfulness, the Buddha simply instructs us to be aware of—without trying to change—conditions of the heart and mind that are particularly significant for our practice of awakening, such as the presence or absence of desire, hatred, ignorance, contraction, and distraction: "When his mind is hating something, the practitioner is aware, 'My mind is hating.' When his mind is not hating, he is aware, 'My mind is not hating.' . . . When her mind is distracted, she is aware, 'My mind is distracted.' When her mind is not distracted, she is aware, 'My mind is not distracted.'" It is the awareness itself—not what may or may not be passing through it—that is most important.

When you're in a conscious and respectful relationship with your emotions, you can respond intelligently to them rather than blindly reacting. And even the darkest can be compost for your spiritual garden. As one Buddhist text, Vimilakirti Nirdesa Sutra, proclaims, "Flowers like the blue lotus, the red lotus, the white lotus do not grow on the ground in the wilderness but do grow in the swamps and mud banks. Just so, the Buddha qualities grow in those living beings who are like swamps and mud banks of passions."

As you become familiar with the labyrinths of your own emotional world, you can embrace the complexities of others'. You can be with the friend who's grieving a spouse who just died without being triggered by your own unacknowledged terror: *What if that happened to me?* You can accommodate a partner's anger or jealousy, having come to terms with your own.

ASANA AND EMOTIONS

Consciously using your yoga asana practice to navigate the stormy surf of your emotions involves a balance of first getting to know your emotional body just as it is and then skillfully working with it to release contraction and encourage positive qualities. This week we'll focus on the first aspect—getting intimate with the emotional body. In week 11 we'll touch on the power of yogic practices to bring about transformation.

The cornerstone of mindfulness of the emotions is the ability to hold whatever is bubbling up in the embrace of your own compassionate attention without needing to fix anything.

Skye's former preschool teacher, a longtime mindfulness practitioner named Leslie Grant, teaches children to sense their heart as an ocean and the emotions as fish swimming through it: *Here comes the anger fish! Now here's the joy fish!* The preschool kids get really excited about this game and especially enjoy running around the room acting out the parts of the various fish. (You may want to try this yourself, although if you make the mistake of doing it at snack time, you are likely to spill your juice box.) This game embodies an important truth: Your emotions, even the ones that are most colorful, are not who you are. They are simply what happens to be swimming through you.

Your mindful asana practice can support this unentangled intimacy with your emotions in several ways.

It increases your capacity to open to strong feelings. Through mindful asana, you've enhanced your ability to be with intense sensations without grasping at them, pushing them away, or ignoring them. Now you can draw on this ability to open to strong emotions as well, even challenging ones.

When the emotional winds start to rise, asana practice provides stability in the nervous system that gives you the confidence to let them howl through you without fearing that you will be blown away. Standing poses keep you rooted in the earth. Back bends familiarize you with opening an armored heart. Forward bends train your body in the art of surrender.

And emotions that might otherwise be overwhelming, such as grief or fear, can be opened to as physical sensations: tightness in the jaw, gripping in the pelvic floor, a knot in the shoulders, heat in the face. When you can be with them simply as sensation, they often become less threatening. You can move out of the story that accompanies these feelings and into the direct experience of them.

It increases your sensitivity. You've practiced the art of tracking even subtle fluctuations of pressure, heat, tension, and release. Now you can use this sensitivity to track your emotions as well—without getting entangled in the stories that accompany them.

Sometimes emotions make themselves known first as a constellation of physical sensations. Resting in a supported back bend, you might notice a pressure in your chest and throat; as you pay attention, it tightens and throbs. You stay with the tightness until it softens and tears begin to flow. Only then do you realize: *I'm really sad.* In a long-held Pigeon Pose, your hips begin to burn. After several minutes, the burning dissolves and you notice a contraction in your pelvic floor. As you soften the pelvic floor, your jaw releases, and suddenly you know: *I'm furious.*

It frees locked emotions. As you open your body, long-buried passions and griefs dislodge from your tissues. More and more of your inner world becomes accessible. This doesn't mean that you need to dredge up the past or work yourself into a frenzy of catharsis. In fact, one of the beauties of an asana practice is that emotions often flow away—in a gale of giggles or a shower of tears—without any need for you to analyze them.

Being Attentive

What transforms an asana practice from physical workout to emotional exploration is where you put your attention. If you do a Wide-Legged Forward Bend with most of your attention on the physical alignment and muscular stretch, that's where most of the transformation will occur. Do the same pose with your attention on the attitude in your heart, and that's where the primary action will be.

Sometimes you can get so obsessed with getting your femur head precisely aligned in its socket that you don't notice the anxiety that's fueling this quest. You're so busy trying to balance in Handstand that you don't notice the self-loathing that surges through you every time you tumble out. You're so fixated on the placement of your hands in a back bend that you don't savor the joy that surges as your heart opens.

Of course, even an asana practice that's primarily physically focused will transform your emotional state, and even a practice that's mainly focused on emotional sensitivity will affect your musculature. But where you place your attention shapes the way your practice unfolds and how it manifests in your life beyond the mat.

And just as with physical sensations, you will learn through paying attention that emotions you thought were immutable—your fear of flying, your affection for your cat—are actually always shifting.

You might tell yourself: *I'm in love.* But does *in love* feel the same at every moment? What about that moment just after breakfast on the first day of your vacation in Bali, when you wanted him to walk hand in hand on the beach with you but instead he pulled out his iPad to read the *New York Times,* which you personally feel that he is addicted to in a somewhat compulsive way? As you steer the U-Haul laden with all of your furniture down the freeway, you might think, *I'm sad to be moving away from this city after fifteen years.* But does that story include the quiver of excitement as you drive away into a new life?

Look closely and the story entitled "I'm in Love" or "I'm Sad" dissolves into a river of unique moments. And this ever-changing flow is much more interesting than any narrative you might solidify around it, just as a trip is richer than the photos you post online when you get back.

In the course of your life, you might walk through arid deserts of grief, when it seems that you will never be happy again. But you will eventually pass through them. And moment by moment, what you thought was solid—such as a pain in your leg—turns out to be fluid. Emotions that you thought lasted for years may only have lasted for fifteen seconds at a stretch in a solid form. It was only the story that stayed the same.

Once you see that, you're less likely to buy in to the reports that your mind is endlessly bellowing. Our stories can get calcified into tracks that the clanking trolley cars of our thoughts trundle over again and again. But the actual scenery that those cars travel through is constantly shifting. So get off the trolley car and look around for a while. Open to the larger view.

POLICING THE EMOTIONS   David Le

David Le is a police officer in Santa Ana, California, and a two-time graduate of Spirit Rock's Mindfulness Yoga Training.

A few years ago, I was investigating an attempted homicide—a sixteen-year-old tried to stab his mother. I went to the hospital to talk to the mother in her hospital bed. The next day I did some follow-up and arrested the sixteen-year-old.

In my job I've been trained in willpower—how to conquer and win. But my practice of mindful yoga has taught me to be able to follow my body sensations and the emotions that go with them.

My job as a police officer was to get a confession from the boy: to have plan A, then plan B, then plan C to outsmart the suspect and put him behind bars for public safety. When I interviewed him, I began to feel the pressure in my chest. My breath was hard, not slow and smooth. I could feel a little pressure in my belly.

From these physical sensations, I realized that I was angry at him. I was prejudging him and looking down on him. My judgment was arising in me. I only saw it because I was in touch with my body. All of a sudden I was able to watch my judgment at the same time that I was talking to the suspect.

Once I saw the judgment, I could disidentify with it. Then a compassionate feeling toward him arose. I slowed down and began to talk to him like one human talking to another, not an officer talking to a suspect. I was able to find spaciousness within me, and he was able to feel spacious in himself. He was able to reflect back and give me a full account of what happened.

He was so identified with the story line of what his mother had done that had made him angry. When I dropped my judgment, after I got all the information that was required by my job as an officer, I was able to focus on helping him. I helped him to switch his attention from the story line to feeling his anger in his body. I was able to give him another method to work with his feelings.

My attitude toward my work has changed because of my yoga practice. Now I'm not trying to change other people or change the circumstances. I'm just trying to work on myself. No matter what kind of call I'm getting—whether it's robbery, domestic violence, a death investigation, assault with a deadly weapon—I just have to get to know myself. I can see my feelings and see if it's appropriate to be with them or to disidentify from them. There's still violence out there. But I'm just trying to work with my own being.

WEEK 9 PRACTICES

This week's practices are not specific asanas or breathing techniques; rather, they are inquiries and ways of paying attention that can help you heighten your awareness of your emotional body. Begin each day's session with Checking In with Your Heart and Mind. Then, if you want a more dynamic physical practice, move into Tracking Your Emotional Body in Asana Flow (page 196); if you want a more restorative practice, try Tracking Your Emotional Body in Long Yin Holds (page 199). Finish with 20 to 30 minutes of seated meditation highlighting mindfulness of the emotions (page 201).

PRACTICE 9.40
Checking In with Your Heart and Mind (5–10 minutes)

In this week's check-in you'll pay particular attention to your emotional state—especially as it's reflected in your physical body.

At the beginning of your practice, spend 5 to 10 minutes in a comfortable sitting, reclining, or standing meditation position doing the guided Checking In with Body, Heart, and Mind meditation from week 5 (page 130). This week, focus especially on the state of your heart. Open to whatever's going on with friendly interest. Sometimes your emotions will be vivid: *I'm excited. I'm anxious. I'm sad.* Other times you may not be feeling much of anything at all, which is also fine.

If your thoughts are spinning, ask yourself whether an emotion might be driving the mental engine. Remember that your emotions may be expressing themselves simply as a pattern of physical sensations:

Not much going on emotionally, but my jaw sure is clenched and all the muscles around my eyes are tight. Sometimes it's only as these physical constrictions begin to release—over the course of a mindful asana practice—that the emotional content will begin to bubble to the surface. So don't be in a rush to figure anything out or fix anything. What matters is that you start your practice by sending a message to the deepest layers of your emotional being: *I am here to listen to you, if you feel like talking.*

If a strong emotion is present, resist getting sucked into the gravitational pull of any accompanying narrative. Instead, locate the emotion as a feeling in your body.

Notice, too, whether you experience this emotion as pleasant or unpleasant. (Just like physical sensations, emotions generally arrive with a feeling tone.) If you're feeling happy or serene, maybe there's an accompanying narrative about what you did to make yourself feel so good—*It's a sign that my spiritual practice is really progressing*—and how you might perpetuate this feeling: *Now I'll do a whole bunch of back bends and open my heart even more!* If you're feeling sad or angry, notice whether you want to push this unpleasant feeling away: *Handstands, that will make me feel better.* Is your mind reciting all the circumstances that led to your sorrow and plotting the strategies that will eliminate it forever?

Remember, you don't need to dredge anything up. Nor do you need to make any uncomfortable feelings or obsessive thoughts go away before proceeding with your asana practice. Just include the subtle shades of what's actually present. Then ground your attention once more in breath and body sensations and move into your day's asana practice.

PRACTICE 9.41
Tracking Your Emotional Body in Asana Flow (30–60 minutes)

A flowing asana practice can bring fluidity to the emotions as well, breaking up stuck patterns and dislodging feelings from your tissues. Holding each pose longer than you usually might gives the emotional body time to unfurl. In this practice you'll flow through a series of dynamic yoga postures—each one held for 2 to 3 minutes—while deliberately heightening your awareness of your emotional body. To support going slower, set a timer at the beginning of your practice to chime at 2- to 3-minute intervals. Hold each posture for the full duration of the time between chimes.

This inquiry can be done in any sequence of asanas, including any standard routine you might regularly practice. But especially when working with the emotional body, it's good not to get locked into a preconceived idea of how your physical practice is going to unfold. Leave room for course changes. Let the unfolding of your emotional body guide the direction of your physical practice, especially when working with emotionally charged regions such as the neck and throat or the pelvic floor. Move with delicacy through that territory. Be prepared to slow down and listen to the voices that begin to speak. You are not trying to get anywhere or get rid of anything. You are making friends with yourself.

Asana Sequence for Tracking Emotions

If you're not sure what to do for practice 9.41, try the following sequence, focusing on the emotional hot spots of neck, shoulders, upper back, hips, and pelvis: Child's Pose, Downward Facing Dog, Low Lunge, Pigeon, Downward Dog, Warrior I, Warrior II, Side Warrior, Triangle, Half Moon Pose, Revolved Half Moon Pose, Revolved Triangle, Pyramid Pose, Downward Facing Dog; repeat Low Lunge–Pyramid Pose sequence on other side; Wide-Legged Standing Forward Bend (with hands interlaced behind back), Squat, Bridge Pose, Reclining Twist, Savasana.

Remember your mantra: Go no faster than you can stay connected to feeling. Even if you're doing a vinyasa practice, linger in and between the poses. Give yourself enough time to drop below the surface.

As you enter each new posture, take the first minute or so to ground your attention in your kinesthetic awareness of your body and breath. Tend to the usual details of alignment.

Then open your lens of awareness to include your emotional body. Note any mental commentary and the emotional tone that accompanies it, just the way you might routinely check the alignment of your neck and spine. Be especially sensitive to feelings of striving, dissatisfaction, competitiveness, or self-judgment. These feelings—generally largely invisible—can be the primary drivers for our practice, motivating what asanas we choose and how we perform them. Don't judge yourself for having them. But do ask yourself: What do they feel like in your body? What would your practice look and feel like if their grip relaxed?

As you stay in the pose longer than you normally might, observe what you feel as you wait for the timer to chime. What do you feel immediately after it does?

Some days you may come into your asana practice already in the throes of a strong emotion or a repetitive thought pattern—say, you're agitated by an argument with your partner or anxious about an upcoming presentation at work or school. If so, acknowledge these feelings: *My back heel is grounded in Warrior Pose, my arms are lifted, and I'm really angry.* But don't get swept away by the story of why you're feeling that way. Keep coming back to the direct experience in your body.

Sometimes emotional content manifests under the radar as a chronic pattern of contraction so habitual we don't even notice it. So with each new posture, scan the physical body's emotional hot spots for tension: your eyes, your jaw, your pelvic floor, your lower belly, the base of your skull, the root of your tongue, the hollow of your throat. Sometimes you may not be aware that an emotion was there until after it lets go. Your forehead softens, your belly releases, and as you are flooded with well-being, you realize: *Oh. I was afraid.*

There's no need to turn your yoga into emotional target practice. Don't dredge up your most painful memories. Just see what's wriggling free inside you as your body moves and breathes.

If nothing particular is going on in your emotional world, stay grounded in your physical sensations and the rhythmic flow of your breath, which naturally regulates your nervous system and emotional body. And remember that whatever you are feeling is likely to change as you move through your practice, without your needing to analyze it. Our emotions are written in sand, not stone, and the waves of our practice can reshape our shores.

PRACTICE 9.42
Tracking Your Emotional Body in Long Yin Holds (30–60 minutes)

Long holds and slow exploration give space for the emotional body to unfurl its cramped wings. For that reason, a meditative sequence of long-held yin poses—holding each one for at least 4 and up to 8 minutes—can be a great way to cultivate the practice of mindfulness of emotions.

Yin Yoga Sequence

It's helpful to choose a sequence of poses beforehand and stick to it. If you can't decide what to do, try the following sequence: supported Back Bend (over a block or bolster), Butterfly Pose, Pigeon Pose, Revolved Pigeon Pose; repeat Pigeon and Revolved Pigeon to the other side; Sphinx, Cobra, Seated Wide-Legged Forward Bend, Seated Wide-Legged Side Stretch (both sides), Reclining Cross-Legged Twist (both sides), Viparita Karani (supported on a block), Savasana.

For each pose, follow this sequence:

1. Set up your physical body with care, tending to the physical details that ensure you will be able to rest in the pose in a meditative way for an extended period of time without injuring joints and ligaments. Then settle down with yourself as if visiting with a dear friend, letting yourself know that you are there to listen.

2. Keeping the lens of your attention wide, sense into the different levels of your being—body, breath, heart, and mind. Just as you did in your opening practice, Checking In with Your Heart and Mind, acknowledge and make space for any strong emotions that may be present.

3. Now let your breath swell into the foreground of your awareness. Track your inhalation all the way down the central channel of the body to the pelvic floor, letting the pelvic floor widen

and soften in response to the downward, outward spread of the diaphragm. Then track the exhalation back to the center of your heart as the pelvic floor and diaphragm release upward. Anchor your attention to the movement of breath and energy between heart and perineum, two powerful gateways to the emotional body. With every inhale, feel the perineum brightening. With every exhale, feel the heart softening.

4. Keep returning your attention to this anchor of your breath. But if you find yourself repeatedly called away by obsessive thinking—especially if you are repeating the same story again and again—check to see if there is an emotion associated with it. Like a shy animal, sometimes the emotional content of a repetitive thought or story does not reveal itself when you hunt for it. Instead, it pokes its furry head out of its burrow only when you take your attention off the story altogether and return to the anchor of your breath. Then the emotional content emerges: *Underneath that obsessive planning, I'm just really frightened. Underneath the recitation of why I'm right and my friend is wrong, I'm sad.*

   If an emotion wells up, recognize and accept it. Often, acknowledging the emotion beneath a repetitive thought stream brings palpable relief—a softening throughout the tissues, as if muscular and fascial tension had been bracing you against feeling what was actually happening. Take some time to get to know the emotion as it lives in your body: heat in the face, pressure in the chest, clenching around the base of the spine. Give it space to move and breathe, without demanding that it depart—and also without getting caught up in the story it might be packed in. Then, when the physical intensity starts to subside, ask yourself: *Am I willing to rest back into my breath wave again?* Coax yourself back to that simple, rhythmic motion of in and out, pelvic floor to heart.

5. When the timer rings, don't rush out of the pose. If you're lost in thought, complete the process above before releasing. Only then move to the next pose. In this way you train your body and nervous system to move deeper and deeper into presence as you shift your body from one meditative shape to another.

You are a scuba diver going down into the coral reefs of your psyche. Wait long enough and all sorts of strange sea creatures will emerge. Some of them are beautiful tropical fish with fluted, flower-like gills and rainbow colors, graceful and delicate. Others are gnarly monsters that crawl out from under rocks waving slimy tentacles.

You are the ocean in which they swim. You have room for them.

In Your Seated Meditation Practice This Week

After your asana practice, come into seated meditation. As in previous weeks, keep your attention anchored primarily in the flow of breath or the tracking of body sensations.

However, this week, if you find yourself *repeatedly* called away—either by a strong emotion or by a repetitive pattern of thinking—let go of your focus on the breath and let the emotion or repetitive story itself be the object of your mindful attention. Turn your attention to look at it directly. Is it an emotion that's summoning you so imperatively? Or if it's a repetitive story or type of story—such as planning or remembering—is there an emotion living beneath its surface, giving it heat?

Don't view this emotional content as a distraction from your meditation; rather, include it in the embrace of your practice. Following the process described in step 4 of the yin sequence in practice 9.42 (page 200), investigate it as a present-moment experience in the body-mind without getting lost in the stories that may accompany it.

Emotions are as natural as pressure in your knee or dampness in the palms of your hands. So don't get caught in fascination with content. Instead, sense yourself as the presence that holds whatever is arising, like a mother rocking a colicky baby. And when the intensity subsides, return your attention to your anchor in body and breath.

In Your Daily Life This Week

Pause periodically throughout your day to assess the state of your heart. What are the unnoticed emotions that might be driving the way you move through your day? What's behind what you're saying or how you are choosing to spend your precious time?

Driving in heavy traffic? Check in with your heart at every red light. Answering your e-mail? Touch in with your emotional body before pressing Send.

Especially take time to reflect when you're in the grip of a strong emotion—which, of course, is when you're least likely to feel like pausing. About to fire off that stressed-out e-mail, copying everyone in your office? Notice the emotion that's surging through you. Feel it in your body. Invite your neck muscles to soften. Let your breath billow through you. Then look at the e-mail again and see if you really want to send it.

RESOURCES

For an in-depth look at how our emotional life plays out in the body, I recommend Peter Levine's book *In an Unspoken Voice: How the Body Releases Trauma and Restores Goodness*. Jack Kornfield's *The Wise Heart* is a guide to Buddhist psychology infused with Kornfield's inimitable blend of storytelling, poetry, and compassionate wisdom. And for an in-depth study of yoga psychology interwoven with compelling personal stories, read Stephen Cope's books *Yoga and the Quest for the True Self* and *The Wisdom of Yoga*.

Your Storytelling Mind

WHEN SKYE WAS EIGHT years old, one of his favorite books was the *Phantom Tollbooth,* by Norton Juster, in which a bored schoolboy named Milo drives a toy car through a toy tollbooth to find himself in a fantastical world where metaphors come to life. Milo is given a tour of the city of Illusions, which is composed of "things that aren't really there that you can see very clearly."

"If something is there, you can only see it with your eyes open, but if it isn't there, you can see it just as well with your eyes closed," explains his guide, Alex (a boy who walks several feet off the ground). "That's why imaginary things are often easier to see than real ones."

The nearby city of Reality, on the other hand, is completely invisible. Once "a beautiful city of fine houses and inviting spaces," it gradually faded away as its inhabitants grew too rushed and distracted to appreciate it. Curiously, no one even noticed: "They went right on living here just as they'd always done, in the houses they could no longer see and on the streets which had vanished, because nobody had noticed a thing." Some former Reality residents moved permanently to Illusions, which is much more beautiful. But as Alex points out to Milo, "It's just as bad to live in a place where what you do see isn't there as to live in one where what you don't see is."

Meditative practice offers the opportunity to wake up from this trance—to move our home back from Illusions to Reality and see both the beauty and the misery that have become invisible to us: corn bread dripping with butter, broken windows on abandoned houses glimpsed through a train window, the drum of rain on a slate roof, a coyote making its way through the burnt gold of a summer meadow.

But in order to do this, we need to look directly not only at the illusory realities we construct through our thoughts but at the very nature of thinking itself.

Each of us has a spell-casting storyteller inside us—a prolific inner blogger who narrates our life, broadcasts our opinions, and entertains us with tales about who we are, what we've done, and what we might do at some time in the future. We endlessly tweet our updates to the only person who's following us—ourself. And the scary thing is, we tend to believe our own PR, whether it's positive or negative, factual or fictitious. Mark Twain once said, "When I was younger I could remember anything, whether it happened or not; but I am getting old, and soon I shall remember only the latter."

This week we'll continue to explore how our yoga practice can return us from the city of illusions back to the living reality of the body. And we'll also use our practice as an opportunity to shine the light of our awareness upon our thoughts, illuminating their nature in the same way we have illuminated the nature of our body, our breath, and our hearts—because mindfulness of thoughts isn't about exterminating them like an infestation of cockroaches. It's about looking deeply enough at them to see their true nature, learning to live with them with a little more grace, and giving ourselves more freedom to choose which thought seeds to water and which to let wither away.

"THE TROUBLE WITH TRIBBLES"

Meditators often go to war with their thoughts. But there's nothing inherently wrong with thinking. Thoughts produced the Taj Mahal, the iPhone, *Hamlet,* Oreos, the Peace Corps, the Declaration of Independence, frozen yogurt, *One Flew Over the Cuckoo's Nest.* On the other hand, thoughts have also led to nuclear weapons, human trafficking, and the destruction of most of the world's old-growth redwoods. We build a prison made of thoughts we were handed in childhood: *I suck at sports. I'm too special to get a job. I'm not as pretty as my sister. I don't deserve to be loved.* And then we lock ourselves into it for the rest of our lives.

As you probably noticed in your practice last week, your thoughts both fuel and reflect your emotions. Your own unconscious narration of your life can shape not just your emotional reality but your behavior. In one fascinating study, reported in Malcolm Gladwell's *Blink*, researchers found that test subjects who were exposed to words such as *Florida, old, gray, wrinkle,* and *Bingo*—scattered randomly throughout what appeared to be a grammar test—walked more slowly (like stereotypical elderly people) when leaving the test room than when they entered it. People who were exposed to words like *bold, rude, disturb,* and *intrude* were far more likely to interrupt the person running the experiment than those who were primed with *yield, patiently, courteous,* and *respect.* Similarly, the messages you give yourself about who you are—*No one loves me; nothing I do works out*—shape not just the way you feel but the way you interact with others and the choices you make. This power of autosuggestion can be turned to your advantage as you choose to water the seeds of thoughts that bring joy as with the cultivation of metta.

And here's one thing you've probably already noticed about thoughts: left to their own devices, they breed like weasels. Do you remember that episode from the original *Star Trek* series, "The Trouble with Tribbles," where the starship *Enterprise* becomes infested with a species of adorable fuzzy animals who unfortunately turn out to be "born pregnant"? Like those Tribbles, every thought carries a future litter. You're sitting peacefully on your zafu in the corner of your living room, enjoying your breath on a rainy day. It feels so good that you decide that you will go on a meditation retreat, but not somewhere rainy—maybe a beach in Thailand, like the retreat your favorite yoga teacher led last year that you couldn't afford. Clearly, in order to advance your spiritual practice, you need to earn more—maybe you should study software design and work for Google. They have offices in France! If you fell in love in France, you'd raise your kids bilingual. Only what if it didn't work out? . . . and suddenly the timer for your meditation session is chiming—but you barely hear it, lost in speculation about custody laws in the European Union.

The Buddhists have a word for this process—*papancha,* or "proliferation," an onomatopoeic word whose popcorn-sounding name hints at the way a tiny handful of thought kernels can explode into a fluffy mountain of tantalizing snacks that it's hard to resist, especially when garnished with emotional butter and salt.

It's understandable how you might wish to escape into your thoughts when life is hard. If you're sitting in traffic school listening to a cop recite the rules about texting and driving, you'd naturally prefer to imagine yourself on a gondola in Venice. But what about when you're kissing your lover and find yourself mentally hunting for a cabbage soup recipe? And when you're munching on papancha, you're lost. You have no capacity either to notice the nature of your thinking mind or to make choices about which thoughts to believe and which to let go of.

How Can Yoga Asana Help?

So how can your yoga asana practice help with this situation?

First of all, on the most basic level, yoga gets you out of your head and into your body; in the words of the pioneering yogini Angela Farmer, it "drains the brain." Your asana practice invites you to move from the chimerical world of your plans, memories, and ideas into the vibrant pulse of your muscles, organs, nerves, and blood. Yoga's physical postures and deep, rhythmic breathing soothe the jangled nervous system and clenched musculature that may be fueling the engine of your compulsive thinking.

The more present you are in your body as you practice, the more effective this thought-busting process is, but frankly, even the most mindless yoga workout will do it to some degree (as will other forms of vigorous exercise). Through targeting pockets of constriction, yoga asanas break up unconscious physical patterns that both reflect and perpetuate the powerful emotions that may underlie the epic sagas you're telling yourself.

For example, the clenched, defensive posture of fear—ingrained in habitual armoring of the neck and shoulders and jaw—sends urgent signals to the nervous system that, in fact, there is something to worry about. The thinking brain then feels obliged to produce elaborate stories about what this threat is and how we can ward it off. Often this primal, posturally encoded fear can lurk behind even the most mundane thoughts, such as the endless recitation of a to-do list.

Yoga practices and breathing techniques snap this feedback loop. Sometimes there's no need to spend hours struggling with your thoughts or figuring out what they are, why you think them, and what ought to be done about them. Just establish a breath rhythm that speaks directly to the autonomic nervous system, telling your ancient reptilian brain that you are safe. Erase the neuromuscular signature of anger or terror or grief. Then the stories will often subside by themselves—or at least, weaken substantially.

But without deeper investigation, asana alone won't free you of the tyranny of your thinking mind. You can become skilled at cranking through even the sweatiest vinyasa while writing a PhD dissertation in your head, following your set routine or the teacher's instructions as mindlessly as you navigate the familiar freeways to work and arrive at your destination with no idea how you got there. Asana practice can also detonate its own papancha explosion, as you compare yourself favorably or unfavorably with other practitioners or obsess about minute anatomical details of alignment.

And just coming back to your body and letting these thoughts go, while powerful, are not enough to bring about freedom. To do that, it's necessary to look more deeply at the nature of the thinking process.

In your asana practice, you can shine the light of your awareness on the narrative that's accompanying your movements and sensations. Who lives in your head as you're practicing? Is it your inner yoga teacher, barking instructions on what to do next (*Okay, now try jumping from Downward Dog to Crow Pose. Go ahead, you can do it!*) and commenting on your performance (*That was totally lame*)? If you actually *are* a yoga teacher, are you rehearsing a future class as you're practicing, storing up interesting insights and tidbits of wisdom—perhaps even wisdom about mindfulness of thinking? Are you comparing your body with how it has been in the past (*It never used to feel like I was doing a forward bend over a bowl of pudding!*) or how you want it to be in the future? You may even catch yourself lost in a story about something that has nothing to do with yoga whatsoever.

And finally, to develop real insight into the nature of thought, it's vital that you spend some time observing your mind while your body is in the relative stillness of a meditation posture. In a dynamic asana practice, it's hard to go on mental autopilot for very long. Sure, you can flow through a familiar vinyasa while mentally repainting your bedroom. But as the poses get more challenging, sooner or later you'll have to bring your mind back to roughly the same location as your body, if only to avoid toppling over in your handstand. That makes asana a limited tool for penetrating more deeply into the nature of the thinking process itself. It's one thing to pay attention to what's present when what's going on is challenging and engaging, like balancing on one leg in Natarajasana. It's a different—and equally important—art to stay alert when your mind doesn't have so much to entertain it.

By including thinking in your mindfulness practice, you'll learn a lot about the unconscious voices that may be shaping your practice and your life. But more important, you'll learn about the nature of thought itself—and how wispy are the stories to which you have been giving so much power.

FREEDOM FROM THOUGHTS: A MINDFUL YOGA STORY
Linda A.

Linda A. teaches mindful yoga in Tucson, Arizona.

My son is an addict. I'm afraid that he is going to die—and he will if he doesn't stop what he is doing. My grandson is living with his mother, but she is bipolar and can't really be a nurturing and patient parent. I am really fearful for his well-being. So I am really scared a lot of the time. If I'm not careful, my mind can just get going and start spinning out all kinds of scary scenarios about what might happen.

But when I am moving and connecting with my breath, my mind doesn't get so lost in all of these scary thoughts. I'm just really present with what's going on in the moment—where my big toe is, the quality of my breath, what I'm feeling in my body. I experience some contentment and joy at being alive and being able to move in all of these different ways. I can connect with a different kind of energy in the midst of this really scary stuff. My practice brings some equanimity. I recognize that most of what happens in life is outside my control, and I can be at ease with that.

Through my practice, I realize that happiness more than anything is a decision that I can make or not make. I land in the peace of being okay with the way things are and then just follow the path, trudging along through the muck and the mud and all the good stuff.

And one of the big things I know from the time that I've been practicing is that this situation is going to change. I don't know how it's going to change, but it's going to change. And just remembering that makes it less heavy.

WEEK 10 PRACTICES

This week start each practice session with Checking In with Your Thinking Mind (below). Then ground your attention through either Feeling Your Roots (page 213) or Pulsing the Perineum (page 214). For an active asana practice, choose either Space between Breaths, Space between Thoughts (page 216), or Observing Your Thoughts in Motion (page 210). Finally, leave 30 to 40 minutes for seated meditation, in which you practice Observing Your Thoughts in Stillness (page 217).

PRACTICE 10.43
Checking In with Your Thinking Mind (5–10 minutes)

In this week's check-in, you'll pay a little extra attention to the state of your thinking mind and how it's affecting your body and emotions.

At the beginning of your practice, spend 5 to 10 minutes in a comfortable sitting, reclining, or standing meditation posture. Do the guided

Checking In with Body, Heart, and Mind practice from week 5 (page 130). This week, after touching in with your body and breath, give particular attention to the stream of your thoughts. Are they white-water rapids? A lazy brook? A still forest pool? Is your inner commentator live-streaming or taking a coffee break? And what's the tone of the broadcast? Excited? Angry? Judgmental?

Don't get in a war with your mind. If your thoughts are exceptionally active, just notice: "Ah. A busy mind is like this." The moment you allow it to be the way it is, you create a little space around your racing thoughts and can remember that they are not who you are.

Open to the possibility that simmering beneath the surface of a mental story may be an emotional brew that bears no logical connection to the content of the thoughts. Remember that emotions may manifest partially—or even entirely—as physical sensations, contractions, or breathing patterns: *I'm not feeling a thing, but my breath sure is shallow and rapid!* So scan your body for patterns of contraction—a clenched jaw, a hardened belly, a lifted shoulder—and invite them to soften. Sometimes a racing mind is accompanied by a feeling of pressure at the top of the skull or even an electrical sensation in the brain itself, as if you could actually feel the neurons firing.

Remember, there's no need to analyze the content of your thoughts, improve them, or make your mind be quiet. You also don't need to stay with the underlying emotions until they're gone or "fixed." You're just taking the current temperature in your mind, like stepping out onto a balcony in the morning to see what the weather is. Everything's going to change anyway, once you start moving and breathing. You just want to know where you're starting.

At the end of your check-in, return your attention to your body and breath. Exhale 10 long, slow breaths, smoothing the texture of the breath like a thread of silk. Dissolve into the space after the exhalation, then let the inhale roll in on its own. Then stay anchored in your body as you proceed into your asana practice.

PRACTICE 10.44
Observing Your Thoughts in Motion (30–60 minutes)

This practice can be done in any pose or sequence of poses: dynamic, yin, or restorative; easy or challenging. If you're not sure what to do, try this: Warm up with a sequence you're familiar with—say, ten Sun Salutation variations, followed by a series of standing poses. Then choose three poses that are challenging for you that you've been meaning to get to but never do. Then finish with a Reclining Twist followed by a Shoulder Stand, Plow, Fish Pose, and Savasana.

But truly—it really doesn't matter what poses you pick. What's important are the three basic steps: set a timer, set an intention, notice your attention.

Set a timer to chime at 5-minute intervals throughout your practice.

Then set an intention to keep returning your attention to the anchor of whatever part of your body is in contact with the ground. If you're doing standing poses, root into the connection of your feet to the earth. In a Plank Pose, feel the pressure into the roots of your fingers and your flexed toes. Lying on your back, sense the touch points of the back of the skull, upper back, sacrum, heels. Of course, your attention will naturally flow to other details of alignment and sensation as you move into each new asana. But no matter how complex the postures, keep returning to your anchors to the earth. Keep these ever-shifting points of contact in the foreground of your awareness.

Each time the timer rings, pause and notice: Where is your attention now? Is it absorbed in the felt sense of this contact with the earth, as you intended? Or is it somewhere else? If you're fully absorbed in the sensations—not commenting on them in your mind but just feeling them—continue on with your practice. If your mind has gone somewhere else, inquire into where it has gone. (If you're in a challenging or transitional pose that you can't hold, it's fine to come out of it and rest in Child's Pose or standing meditation while you do this inquiry; otherwise just stay in the posture while you inquire.) Don't take too long or get caught in elaborate analysis—that just means more thought proliferation. Just notice what's going on.

- When the bell rang, was your attention resting primarily in sensation or in verbal commentary?
- If you were thinking, were you thinking about your yoga practice—even, perhaps, about the instructions about thought? Were you giving yourself instructions about whatever pose you were in? Or were you thinking about something else entirely?

- Were you thinking in words? Pictures? Music?
- If words, was the voice friendly? Bossy? Angry? Were you pointing out what you were doing wrong or what you were doing right? Whose voice was it?
- Were you planning? Remembering? Rehearsing?
- What happens when you turn to look directly at your thoughts? Do they persist or melt away? Do they change?

If it's helpful, give your thoughts a one-word label: *Planning. Lecturing. Fantasizing.* Then proceed with your practice until the timer chimes again.

Echo Chamber Effect of the Mind

If you're not solidly grounded in your body, examining the nature of your thoughts can feel like being inside an echo chamber—or like standing in a house of mirrors, with infinite versions of yourself stretching away in all directions. You're looking at your thoughts and noticing them—but isn't the inner instruction *Notice your thoughts* also a thought? Isn't that your inner meditation teacher? And isn't the thought *That's my inner meditation teacher* also a thought? If you feel as if you're tapping yourself on the shoulder and spinning around trying to look at your own face, just relax. Return to your body. Ground yourself again and again in the felt sense of breath, of body sensations, just as you've been practicing all along.

And if you notice that you've been swept away by a river of thoughts, take a moment to celebrate: no matter how long you've been gone, now you're back! You're no longer floating down the Ganges in an imaginary canoe or having great sex with an imaginary lover. You're in a forward bend, your hamstrings are tight, your mat smells like dirty socks, and your nose itches. Not so exciting as what you were thinking about, perhaps, but it has one huge advantage: it's actually happening. So celebrate this moment of returning rather than berate yourself for being gone. Welcome yourself home with open arms. That way you're more likely to want to come back.

PRACTICE 10.45
Feeling Your Roots (10 minutes)

Yoga allows you to drop attention away from the cawing of the thoughts in your head and into the grounding earth beneath your feet. From this rooted place you can choose more intentionally—and heartfully—which of your thoughts you want to feed with your attention and which you want to let flutter away.

So if you noticed in your Checking In with Your Thinking Mind—or as you started to flow through your asana practice—that your mind was particularly agitated or scattered, try this variation on standing meditation, which I first learned from Angela Farmer.

Settle into your standing meditation posture (page 145). Find your balanced alignment around your energetic center line. Bring particular attention into the soles of your feet and the felt sense of your connection with the ground.

Now sense into the origins of your legs, deep in your body. Do your legs begin where your thigh bones meet your pelvis? Or can you imagine that they begin even farther up, deep in your belly and lower back? Imagine that, from the deep source of your legs in the back of your belly, tendrils of energy are beginning to sprout. They travel down the backs of your legs, through your ankles, and out the center point of your heel where it connects with the ground beneath you. Then they reach beyond your body—down, down, down into the earth itself. See how deep into the earth you can allow these energetic roots to extend.

As you imagine your roots reaching down, you may feel yourself settling your attention a little more fully into your back body, opening and widening the back to receive your breath as your roots reach farther and farther into the soil. Allow your body to receive and respond to this imagery for a minute or so. As you sense the back of your body and the imaginary roots going down from your heel, feel into the movement of the breath in your nostrils. Where in your nostrils do you sense it most vividly? The front? The sides? Or the back?

Now imagine another set of roots dropping down from your belly right through the core of your legs, through your feet, and down through the ball of your big toe into the earth. Sense these roots, too, spiraling their way down into the ground. Feel and receive this imagery. Now where do you feel the breath in your nostrils?

In a similar way, drop down roots from the balls of the little toes. With each root, sense into the place in your body where the root originates. Observe where you feel the breath moving in your nostrils: To the back? The sides? The front? The center? Feel the arches of the feet lifting to receive the earth energy while all around them the roots reach deeper and deeper. Stand for 10 to 15 minutes, feeling into your connection to the earth.

Going further. From this place of rootedness, think about something. That's right: *Think!* Pick one of the countless mental bones you've been gnawing on. Chew on it a bit while simultaneously being aware of your roots going down into the earth. What is the quality of your attention now? What is the quality of your thinking? Can you think about this topic while simultaneously sensing your roots in the earth?

After a few minutes, let go of the thoughts and return your attention to your roots again.

You can explore going back and forth like this a few times—thinking and rooting, thinking and rooting. See how this changes your relationship to your thoughts.

Variations. This practice can also be done in the seated position. Instead of rooting through your legs and feet, send the roots done from the right and left buttock bones, from the tailbone and inner wall of the sacrum, and from the inner wall of the pubic bones. You can also practice rooting in any of the more dynamic standing postures, such as Warrior or Trikonasana, although you will not be able to hold these poses for as long.

PRACTICE 10.46
Pulsing the Perineum (10 minutes)

◀)) For a guided audio version of this practice, go to www.shambhala.com/movingintomeditation.

Another powerful way of grounding yourself in relationship to the gyrations of your thinking mind is by consciously channeling your attention into the pelvic floor—in particular into the perineum, the triangle of muscle located just between the anus and the genitals. The delicate and sensitive web of tissue is known to yogis as the blossom of the muladhara chakra, the energy wheel that flowers forward from its root in the tip of the tailbone. The root chakra, in yogic psychology, is often linked to feelings of security, groundedness, and safety. And whether or not you believe this correlation between the energy body and the psyche, you may find that moving your attention into this part of the body—and connecting intimately with the felt sense of its subtle pulsation—is a powerful way to draw your attention away from the scampering gerbils in your head.

As we explored in weeks 3 and 4, the pelvic floor and the perineum naturally pulse with the breath, opening, widening, and descending with every inhalation in a movement that mirrors that of the respiratory diaphragm, and then lightly lifting and gathering in with every exhalation. If you have difficulty sensing your pelvic floor moving with your breath, begin exploring your breath in Child's Pose (part 1 of Where Does the Breath Move? in week 3, page 85). Rest here, inviting your pelvic floor to soften until you can feel the perineum blossoming open with the inhale and softening inward with the exhale.

Now sit comfortably in your seated meditation posture with your eyes closed. As you inhale, let your breath draw your attention in and down. Sense the soft palate softening and widening, the diaphragm moving down, and the pelvic floor releasing and widening. As you exhale, sense the pelvic floor and the perineum gathering in and up, the diaphragm lifting, and the soft palate slightly doming.

Keep spiraling your attention down and in until it rests right in the center of your perineum. Live inside this subtle pulsation. Remember, this isn't a motion you have to create. It's an undoing rather than a doing. Just keep sensing the flower opening with every inhalation, closing slightly with every exhalation. You also might imagine the perineum brightening slightly with every inhalation and dimming with every exhalation.

Sit for 5 to 10 minutes, relaxing into this movement. Notice what this does to your relationships with your thoughts.

Going further. You can intensify this energetic action by adding a deliberate *mula bandha,* or root lock—the slight lifting and toning of the pelvic floor and the perineum. Often taught forcefully as a contraction of the anus or the vaginal muscles, it can be felt more subtly—and ultimately more powerfully—as a delicate lift, as if tugging upward on the center of a spiderweb. As you inhale, glide your attention down the breath as the perineum expands. As you exhale, lightly engage your mula bandha, drawing up on the perineum. Keep your attention in the feeling of the perineum lifting through the duration of the exhalation. Then release the mula bandha and let the breath swell back in, the perineum widening. At the top of the inhale, pause for just a heartbeat, rooting your attention in the tip of the tailbone. Then exhale as you engage your mula bandha again.

Repeat for 10 rounds, then release the practice. Let your attention rest again in the natural movement of the breath in the pelvic floor. Again, notice your relationship with your thoughts.

PRACTICE 10.47
Space between Breaths, Space between Thoughts (10–15 minutes)

Like your breath, your thoughts arise out of nothing and dissolve back to nothing. So heightening your awareness of the space between thoughts can be a powerful way of freeing yourself from their grip. And heightening your awareness of the space between breaths can help you do that.

Revisit the practices in week 4 that explore the pause between breaths (practices 4.19, 4.20, and 4.21, on pages 102–6). Pay particular attention to what happens to your thoughts in those pauses. Notice how the breath arises out of empty space and dissolves back into that space again. Can you see how thoughts do the same?

Then explore the following more-dynamic and active version of that practice, which I learned from the yoga therapist Janice Gates. Take a simple, dynamic sequence of yoga postures that you know well. For instance, a simple Sun Salutation or a repetitive flow through a sequence of standing postures (Warrior I, Warrior II, Side Warrior, Triangle, Revolved Triangle; back to Warrior I). Flow through it first with a steady, comfortable breath pattern: inhaling 5 counts, exhaling 5 counts. Then begin to open out the space between breaths. First flow through the sequence while suspending the breath for 1 count when the lungs are empty and then again when the lungs are full, like this: inhale 5, pause 1, exhale 5, pause 1. Repeat the sequence four more times, each time extending the pause 1 count longer. The cycle is complete when the rhythm is an equal ratio: inhale 5, pause 5, exhale 5, pause 5.

As you flow, relax into the lengthening pauses between breaths. Notice what happens to your thoughts on the full pause and the empty pause. Is it different?

After you've completed this sequence, sit, stand, or lie down and just rest in stillness, observing the natural flow of your breath.

In Your Seated Meditation Practice This Week

This week be sure to set aside at least 30 to 40 minutes for your seated or standing meditation. However you arrange your body, the basic practice is the same: Rest your attention on whatever anchor point you've chosen in your breathing body. And then notice the kinds of journeys your thoughts try to take you on.

One popular approach that aids in this process is to imagine that you are seated in the shade of a tree on the bank of a beautiful river watching the sun sparkling off the ripples as the waters flow by. Bobbing past you are the boats of your thoughts, with their bright and captivating sails. All you have to do is relax and watch them go by. But again and again, without quite knowing how it has happened, you find that you've gotten on a boat.

One of these boats might be a Planning boat, full of people fretting and worrying about their upcoming job applications, their grocery lists, their taxes. One of them is probably a Romance boat, where everyone is kissing and holding hands and gazing misty-eyed into the sunset. One of them is a Regret boat, where everyone hashes over her or his biggest mistakes again and again. Once you're on a boat, you're immediately swept up into whatever is going on there.

But here's the thing—as soon as you realize you're on the boat, all you have to do is fly back to your seat on the riverbank. Relax your body. And continue to watch the boats go by.

Try this visualization and see if it helps you. But don't get obsessive about it. Think too much about it and suddenly you're on another boat—the Thinking about Meditation boat. So hop off that one too. Return to the riverbank and reconnect with the anchor of your body and breath.

Going further. With most thoughts, it's enough just to notice them and let them dissolve, returning your attention again and again to your anchor in your body and breath. Some of them, however, are more persistent. What if there's a particular boat that you find yourself boarding again and again and riding for miles?

In that case, here are a few helpful inquires:

- Just as you did in Checking In with Your Thinking Mind, notice whether there's an emotion that underlies the persistent thought or story. If so, your goal is not to get rid of it but to take good care of it, as you might care for a bird with a broken wing. Once you tend to the emotion that's fueling the thought, the shouts of the storytelling mind—which was trying so hard to capture your attention—often subside. Knowing that you're angry and feeling it in your body as it manifests right now is not the same as being on the Anger boat, your bags all packed, carried off down the river.

- Name the boats that you board most frequently. Are you especially fond of the Blame boat? The Career boat? Maybe you like to get on the Yoga boat; this is a popular one, especially for yoga teachers: *How will I give instructions for this particular pose? How will I talk about this particular insight?* Once you know what boats you prefer, you may catch yourself as you're about to step on the gangplank. You may even see their sails approaching way down the river and know that you can just wave and let them float on by.

  Particularly with those favorite boats, your mind will come up with lots of good reasons why it's really important that you get on board. *I'm afraid my child might be autistic. That sculpture I've been struggling with—I just had a great idea for how to mix the clay! If I don't think about this right now then . . . then . . .* Then what? Notice the emotion that comes up when you really loosen your grip on the thought's handle. That's the emotion that was fueling it.

- Pay attention to the fundamental energy—beneath even the emotional content—that's powering the thoughts. Is your story line fueled by grasping for something you don't have? Is it fueled by aversion: you are either pushing something away in anger or contracting from it in fear? Is it fueled by delusion, an attempt to keep some personal identity propped up like a Halloween scarecrow? Or are your thoughts fueled by the energy of love, compassion, generosity, and gratitude? See how these energies manifest as felt sensations in your body. Through your mindful yoga practice you have been honing your ability to track the subtle fluctuations of sensation and energy throughout your body. Now is your chance to reap the benefits of this training.

- Notice what form your thinking takes. Do you think in pictures? In stories? Do most of your thoughts consist of conversations with people in which you are describing your experiences and insights? Do you see your thoughts spelled out like a news crawl? As your attention gets more stable and refined, notice the insubstantial nature of thoughts themselves—how they arise out of nowhere, unbidden; how they dissolve into nothingness again. In my hometown in the summer a man with a giant bubble wand hangs out in a roadside park, creating bubbles as big as cars. Some of them drift into the road, and several times I've driven right into one of them. No matter how big they are, they still pop into just a few spatters of soap as soon as the front bumper hits them.

  That's how it is with the thoughts, too. Even the biggest ones pop like soap bubbles into a little spatter of soap and air. Think about the top ten thoughts you were obsessed by—consumed by—ten years ago. Can you even remember them? Sooner or later, the clenched fist of your mind will be forced to release even the things it clings to most tightly. So it's good to learn to do it voluntarily.

In Your Daily Life This Week

As you go through your days, notice what kinds of thoughts draw you away from the present moment. Are you usually planning for the future? Replaying the past? What are the top five movies playing in your inner theater this week? Are they horror films or romantic comedies? What version of you is starring in them? But most of all, pay attention to the moment when your thought bubbles pop and you return to the reality of the moment: stirring a pot of simmering soup, sitting in your car at a red light opposite a grocery store. In those moments, as your seemingly solid fantasies reveal themselves as the flimsy facades they truly are, how do you feel?

Meditation and Creative Thinking

I often teach at the annual Spirit of Creativity retreat at Spirit Rock, which combines meditation, yoga, painting, and writing. A room that's normally reserved for walking meditation is turned into a painting studio, and over the course of the silent week, walls hung with blank white sheets of paper blossom into a blazing garden of color and shapes—goddesses, demons, bloody-toothed flowers, multicolored vaginas, eagles bursting from dark caves with snakes writhing from their talons. It's as if a nuclear bomb has gone off in a dream factory, scattering hallucinatory pieces of unconscious imagery all over the walls. Meanwhile, on the sun-scorched hills, writers sit under trees and on rocks scribbling furiously in notebooks or tapping away at laptops and tablets, spinning out poems, plays, stories, and visions.

This magnificent explosion of creativity is punctuated by long periods of silent sitting and walking meditation. So it's inevitable that the question comes up among the retreatants: *Why should I be turning my attention back to my breath and body when I'm having so many great creative ideas?* You are sitting by a river leaping and flashing with the backs of idea fish: poems surfacing, then vanishing; the looming mass of a novel visible under the surface, only its dorsal fin protruding from the water. How can you let all of these great ideas swim by? Shouldn't you cast in your net?

Actually, meditation can be a powerful support for the creative process. It cultivates your ability to choose where you put your attention rather than being helplessly yanked this way and that. Your growing ability to return your attention again and again to your chosen anchor—for instance, breath or body sensations—will serve you well when you do choose to catch one of those creative ideas in your net. As a writer, the sensitivity and focus you are developing will help you listen to the faint voices of the characters who are trying to make their way into your story. As a painter, it will enable you to notice the images that want to pour through you that may not be the ones you think you ought to paint. Meditation training will give you the persistence to continue with your creative journey even when your inner hecklers are booing and throwing tomatoes (or worse still, helpfully pointing out that your creation is nothing compared to the work of the great masters and you should stop wasting your time.)

While some of the thoughts you have during meditation are truly brilliant, many of them are like the notes you scrawl on scraps of paper in the middle of the night about the brilliant insights you had in your dreams, which upon waking say something like: *What about selling single socks on eBay?* The mind is a fountain of creativity, spewing out seeds like a dandelion scatters fluff. Most of them won't land and plant, and that's okay; there are more than enough. The best ideas, the ones that are really worth pursuing, will still be there when you leave your meditation and pick up your pencil or paintbrush. They'll knock on your door again and again, demanding that you give yourself to them. And the more wholly you've surrendered to breath and body in meditation, the more wholly you'll be able to surrender to the creative flow.

I started writing my first published novel when my son was four and didn't finish until he was seven. As I dove deeper and deeper into it, I realized I was in danger of sacrificing my actual life—the one where I had a child, a job, an ex-husband, a series of boyfriends—for the imaginary life of my character. I was sautéing summer squash and white beans while thinking about Amanda wandering through India: Would she have her baby at an ashram? Or return to her boyfriend in the States? I was hiking with a dear friend through a field of purple lupine, fretting about Amanda's adventures at a tantra party in Khajuraho. So I made a rule for myself: as I wrote my novel, I would write only when I was *actually writing.* That didn't mean that my mind didn't wander to my novel's plot as I was at a farmer's market under the redwoods, sniffing the stem end of cantaloupes to see if they were ripe. It just meant that whenever I caught it, I would let go of my ideas—no matter how good I thought they were—and return to the moment: placing the cantaloupe in my cloth shopping bag while listening to a blind musician with a wreath of flowers and fruit in her hair sing "Puff, the Magic Dragon." I learned to trust that when I sat down at my keyboard the next morning and opened the gates of my unconscious, whatever had been storing up there would come galloping, creeping, hobbling, or dancing out and onto the page.

RESOURCES

For a clear presentation of mindfulness of thinking, check out the classic *Mindfulness in Plain English* by Bhante Gunaratana or *Fully Present: The Science, Art, and Practice of Mindfulness* by Susan Smalley and Diana Winston. For more practice "draining the brain" and rooting into the earth, look to the guided imagery of Angela Farmer and Victor van Kooten, as beautifully illustrated in Victor's book *From Inside Out.*

Weeding the Garden

IT IS A RAINY March day, and my friend Mia is helping me in my neglected winter garden—digging out dead tomato plants and bitter celery, spreading mulch, rescuing the rosebushes from a fungus caused by my forgetting to turn off the irrigation through the rains.

Mia is an organic gardener and a wild-food forager—the sort of person who will leach the tannins out of acorns, roast them, and grind them up to make acorn-flour cookies in the way of the ancient Miwok who used to inhabit this coastal valley. (I, on the other hand, am the sort of person who might buy acorn-flour cookies at the health food store, eat two of them in the car, and then lose the rest in a drift of unsorted mail in the passenger seat in the way of the modern Multitaskers who inhabit this coastal valley now.)

Five or six years ago, Mia used my garden as the subject of her year-long final project in permaculture school. Over the course of a year, Mia tracked patterns of shade, sunlight, wind, rainfall, and runoff. She noted where I practiced yoga on summer mornings and where Skye liked to read in the shade of an oak. She mapped our regular routes from kitchen to compost, car to mailbox.

At the end of the year, she drew a beautiful map of the whole property in colored pencil. It included all the information she had gathered about the current state of the garden. But it also included ways we might want to develop it: the best place to plant a peach tree, raspberry patch, or herb garden; where we might place rainwater reclamation barrels or shore up an eroding hillside.

Working with Mia in the garden, I am reminded that this is what it can be like to tend the acreage of the human heart and mind. First you spend some time getting to know its wild nature: Where are the tangles of brambles and blossoms? Where do the long shadows of anger and anxiety tend to fall? You run your fingers through the mental and emotional soil, assessing its texture: rich and fertile in some places, gritty or clay-like in others. But you don't just sit there studying it forever. Once you're familiar with your little plot of land, you can begin to pull up weeds, fertilize the soil, and plant fruit and flowers.

Over the past two weeks, you've been training your ability to greet your emotions and thoughts with loving awareness and without judging or trying to change them. But being mindful doesn't mean that you are simply a passive observer. In his teachings on the fourth foundation of mindfulness, the Buddha asks us to investigate and see for ourselves: Which habits of the heart and mind—and what way of perceiving the world around us—support wisdom, joy, and awakening, and which ones lead to further suffering? What are skillful means to encourage the mind states that point us toward liberation and mitigate the ones that keep us ensnared?

Of all the different weeds that grow in the garden of our heart and mind, the Buddha pointed to five common varieties that are most likely to crowd out the blossoms and fruit of joy and happiness. Known in Buddhist psychology as the Five Hindrances, they're likely to show up again and again in your meditation and your life, blocking your access to your innate wisdom and kindness. They are traditionally identified as craving, aversion, sloth and torpor, restlessness, and doubt.

I like to think of these hindrances as the Five Opportunities—because each one points to a place where we can reconnect with our capacity for loving presence. They aren't just roadblocks to our inner journey; they are the road itself. I don't know anyone truly wise and compassionate who hasn't gotten there by facing and working through at least one (and probably more) of these painful (and human) tendencies.

This week we'll investigate how a mindful yoga practice can help us understand and transform each of these five energies as well as nourish the blossoming of positive qualities to replace them. To structure your practice, first read through the descriptions of all the hindrances and the practices that accompany them. Then choose your practice each day based on which obstacle feels most active in your psyche. If you're in doubt, begin with half an hour of seated meditation and see what distracts you. And if you're in the happy situation of having no obstacles to your calm, clear, relaxed presence, then just choose one hindrance each day to investigate. That way you'll have the appropriate practices in your tool kit when you need them.

WEEK 11 PRACTICES

Opportunity 1: Craving

Classically listed as the first—and most problematic—of the Five Hindrances, craving is the feeling you might get as you walk through the merchandise-strewn foyer of a yoga studio and are suddenly consumed by the need to purchase an om anklet, a Himalayan salt lamp, a pashmina shawl, and panties printed with the seven chakra symbols. It's the compulsive feeling of wanting *more, more, more, more,* whether it's ice cream, approval, coffee, sex, money, fame, or any of the other lures the world dangles.

You might specialize in cravings for things: the latest smartphone, designer shoes. Your craving of choice might be experiences: a trip to Italy, a soak in a hot tub. You might pine for a new identity as, say, a famous actor or writer or musician. In your yoga practice, craving might manifest as the longing for a deeper back bend, more flexible hamstrings, or a romance with the yogi on the next mat. Craving can be intense and overwhelming, as with romantic obsession. Or it can be a subtle but pervasive background sense of wishing for something other than what's actually happening.

However it shows up, craving is painful. It's a whimper or a shriek from a part of you that doesn't feel whole the way you are. Craving whines *This isn't enough.* And since, at any given moment, *this* is all there is, craving can never be satisfied—like the hungry ghosts who wander through Buddhist mythology, their necks too thin to pass food through to their immense, insatiable stomachs.

It's wonderful to savor and celebrate the many pleasures of human life. In fact, as you've probably experienced, yoga asana practice can heighten sensual pleasure: food tastes better, music sounds more beautiful, sex becomes more passionate and satisfying. Asana practice springs from the tantric tradition of yoga, which is all about using the body as a vehicle of awakening. And as one Buddhist tantric text (the Candamaharosana Tantra) puts it:

> To renounce the sense objects
> Is to torture oneself by asceticism—don't do it!
> When you see form, look!
> Similarly, listen to sounds,
> Inhale scents,
> Taste delicious flavors,
> Feel textures.
> Use the objects of the five senses—
> You will quickly attain supreme Buddhahood.

But as we explored in week 8, mindfulness practice asks us to look at where we're *hooked* on pleasant experiences—where we're not merely enjoying something but believe that our happiness depends upon it. It's that sticky, compulsive quality that turns the life-affirming pleasure of sensuality into the torture of craving. It's what advertisers count on evoking when they bombard you with images of blissful, beautiful people consuming their products. And much of what the world invites you to chase after is what I once heard Thich Nhat Hanh call "plastic bait"—it looks tasty but will not nourish you deeply. As he said, "In plastic bait, there is always a hook."

Responses

So what do you do when craving seizes you? For all of the hindrances, it's helpful to begin with the simple process for meeting difficult mind states that is often known to contemporary Western Buddhist teachers by the acronym RAIN:

1. *Recognize* (R) that craving is present. Name it for what it is: *Oh. This is craving.* Sometimes just naming a hindrance when you notice it arising can give you a little freedom from its grip on your heart.
2. *Accept* (A) that it's there. Don't be at war with your own mind. This doesn't mean that you have to like it. It just means that you're acknowledging with kindness the truth of how things are right now.
3. *Investigate* (I) it. What does craving feel like? Where does it live in your body: A tightness in the chest or belly? A pressing of the tongue against the roof of your mouth? A quickened breath? Break your focus on the object of your desire—the fudge brownie, the hybrid car—and get really curious about the actual experience of craving itself.
4. *Nonidentify* (N). Remember, as you experienced last week, that you are larger than whatever emotion is blowing through you. You are the ocean that the great white shark of craving is swimming through. You are not the toothy, hungry jaws.

In this four-step process, you draw on all the skills you've been deepening over the past 10 weeks for tracking the state of your body, breath, mind, and heart without judging or getting mired in them. Getting to know a hindrance in this way—without going to war with it—is the most important part of freeing yourself from its tyranny.

Once you've used the RAIN process to get familiar with the state of your inner garden, you can—like a skilled horticulturist—begin to work it with the tools from your yogic toolshed. For each hindrance, there are particular yogic practices—based in the physical body—that can help you find your way back to your essential wholeness. Remember, these are not magic bullets. They are somatic tools for loosening the grip of a hindrance on your body and mind, so you can see more clearly its nature—and your own.

When struggling with craving, practice the art of enjoying pleasant sensations without hanging on to them (A Few of Your Favorite Things, page 183). Another powerful tool is the yogic technique of *pratyahara,* or sense withdrawal—withdrawing the senses from their fixation on the outer world and turning them inward to find a source of delight that is not dependent upon whether we satisfy all of our desires. The Turning the Senses Within practice, which follows, is a simple way to develop pratyahara.

PRACTICE 11.48
Turning the Senses Within (10 minutes)

In this practice you temporarily withdraw your senses from the tantalizing stimulation of the outside world to reconnect with your inner balance and tranquillity. The audible pranayama known as Bee Breath heightens the internal focus.

Rest in any reclining restorative pose. (If you're not sure what to do, I recommend a simple and soothing Legs Up the Wall: lie on your back with your sit bones near the wall and your legs stretched upward, resting against the wall's support.) Cover your eyes with an eye pillow and block your ears with earplugs. Or, wrap a cloth bandage snugly around your head so it covers both eyes and ears.

Soften your sense gateways: your skin, your inner ears, your jaw and tongue, your nostrils. With the eyes closed, turn your inner gaze downward toward the heart. Imagine that you are seeing, hearing, and sensing your interior world rather than the world around you. Dive deep inside.

Now connect with the whisper of your breath in and out. After a natural inhale, exhale with a humming sound, touching the lips together and making the sound of the letter *M* for the duration of the exhalation: *Mmmmmmmmmm*. Then inhale normally and repeat.

With the ears plugged or covered, the humming sound will reverberate through your skull. Become absorbed in its hypnotic buzz. The longer your exhalations, the more compelling and soothing the sound will be—but don't strain. Let the exhalations deepen on their own.

Practice Bee Breath for as long as is comfortable, up to 5 minutes. Then return to resting in your natural breath for a few more minutes. Before coming out of your pose, notice: Do the sensations of craving still dominate your body?

Opportunity 2: Aversion

You're three days into a yoga retreat you've been looking forward to for months, and everything is bugging you, from the vegan dinners to the tropical sun to the teacher's choice of music (you are *so over* Sanskrit hip-hop). How can paradise be such hell?

The flip side of craving, aversion—sometimes translated as ill will or hatred—manifests as pulling away from or lashing out at something or someone we don't like, whether it's the weather, a politician, or the perfume worn by the woman on the next mat. As you experienced in week 8, it's a natural human response to an unpleasant sensation—and it can range from a low-grade, grumbling dissatisfaction to full-blown rage, hatred, or terror.

In your yoga practice you might see aversion arising as a dislike of a particular teacher, style of yoga, or sequence of postures. Or it might manifest as discontent with your body, especially as compared with the bodies around you. Sometimes it's so pervasive that it is almost invisible, the unexamined motive for almost everything you do: *I'm not good enough, I need to change. This situation isn't right, I'd better fix it. This person is wrong. That point of view is bad.* When its flames burn unchecked, they can grow to the wildfires of violence, murder, and war. You can do things you regret for the rest of your life.

Responses

As with all of the hindrances, if you're having an aversion attack, the first thing to do is go through the RAIN process. Recognize and accept that aversion is there. Feel into where your anger or fear might live in your body—especially tuning in to their common reservoirs in the jaw, belly, and pelvic floor. Without labeling them as wrong, is there a way you can invite these areas to soften, or at least that you can soften around them?

Return to week 8 and revisit how to open to unpleasant experiences without pushing them away or contracting. (And remember that sometimes the experiences we most resist are the ones that bring us the greatest gifts.)

A classic antidote to aversion is metta practice. So return to week 7 for a refresher and try sending a little metta to the situation or person that's triggering your irritation (Metta Blooming, on page 165). Finally, one of the most potent antidotes to aversion is gratitude. The Buddha often instructed monks and nuns to cultivate gratitude by going into the woods, sitting at the base of a tree, and "gladdening the heart" by reflecting on all the circumstances that made possible this precious opportunity to practice the path of awakening. The Buddha's emphasis on this practice hints that twenty-five hundred years ago, as now, the human and even the monastic tendency was to notice what's wrong rather than what's right. So try the following gratitude meditation.

PRACTICE 11.49
Gratitude Meditation (10–30 minutes)

Your mind responds to specifics more vividly than to generalities, as any poet knows. So be as precise in articulating gratitude as possible: not just general gratitude for having enough to eat but specific gratitude for the hot oatmeal with cinnamon and bananas you ate for breakfast. Not just gratitude for your friends but for Carole's laughter and Spencer's knobby knees and the way Sienna fills her home with the smell of baking apples.

Come to a comfortable seated, standing, or reclining meditation position. Then, one at a time, conjure up and reflect on 5 to 10 things you're thankful for.

You may find you return to some favorites every day. But also challenge yourself to come up with at least 4 or 5 new gratitude objects in each meditation. You may be astonished how much you have to be thankful for.

Linger on each image for at least 5 full breaths, amplifying the gratitude with each inhalation and infusing it throughout your whole body on each exhalation. If it helps, you can verbally note it with each breath: *As I breathe in, I am grateful for the peach I had for breakfast. . . . As I breathe out, I appreciate the hard work of the organic farmer who grew it.* Or if words feel distracting, just stay with the direct feeling of gratitude.

As with any meditation practice, you're likely to catch your mind wandering or returning to its ingrained habit of noticing what's wrong: *Sure, that salad was great. But then I ate two slices of tiramisu and stayed up past midnight . . . now I feel bloated and exhausted.* That's okay. As soon as you catch yourself, thank your mind for all the thoughtful (or thought-full) ways it tries to look out for you. Release any temptation to get lost in a proliferation of thoughts about what you're grateful for (and how you might make those things even better or get more of them). You may even want to take a moment to use your mind itself as the object of your gratitude meditation: *Breathing in, I'm grateful for my ever-creative mind, with its fountain of useful ideas. . . .*

When you have contemplated 5 or 10 gratitude objects, let go of the specific objects and invite the general feeling of gratitude that you have invoked to infuse your whole body. Don't try to coerce yourself: if you don't feel grateful, just notice that. But till the soil and plant the seeds so gratitude can flower when it's ready.

Opportunity 3: Sloth and Torpor

This quaintly named hindrance manifests as sleepiness, lethargy, or a lack of energy for (or interest in) your yoga and meditation practice. If every time you hit the cushion your head starts nodding, or if you find yourself dragging leaden limbs from one asana to the next, you might be having a sloth-and-torpor attack.

Like all the hindrances, this is a normal human condition that doesn't necessarily vanish with advanced practice. On one meditation retreat, I heard two monks exchanging sleepiness stories. One recounted falling asleep not just while listening to a dharma talk but while *giving* one. The other told of dozing off while leading a meditation session, then tumbling forward and ringing the bell with his forehead.

Responses

If you're struggling with this obstacle, spend a little time investigating where it springs from. Are you just exhausted? Many people come to meditative practice deeply worn out from stressful and overcommitted lives. If that's the case, you might need to replenish your well with some supported restorative yoga poses or even a long nap.

Are you drifting off to sleep because you're avoiding a difficult emotion or thought that's trying to bubble up? If so, clear some space for it to emerge into consciousness.

However, it might just be that your balance of energy and tranquillity—two essential components of meditative practice—is out of whack. Too much energy and you'll be agitated and restless; too much tranquillity and you'll doze off. Fortunately, yogic techniques can help restore you to relaxed alertness.

As you learned in week 4, yoga teaches us to move fluidly and at will between activating the sympathetic and parasympathetic nervous systems. The sympathetic nervous system is the accelerator of the body-mind system—it prepares the body for fight-or-flight action via a synchronized marshaling of resources that includes diverting blood from the digestive organs to the muscles, cuing the adrenal glands to pour out the natural stimulant of adrenaline, and raising the heart rate. The parasympathetic nervous system is the brake—it soothes the nerves, down-pedals the adrenal flow, slows the heart, and prepares the organs to rest and digest.

Yogic practices—especially pranayama—enable us to activate one system or the other intentionally. We can stimulate the sympathetic nervous system through strong muscular action and rapid breathing. We can stimulate the parasympathetic nervous system through muscular relaxation, slow breathing, and inversions.

So if you're feeling sluggish, go for the wake-up asanas that activate the sympathetic nervous system, such as back bends and handstands. (Iyengar's prescription for depression was to "open your armpits.") Choose pranayama practices that emphasize the inhalations. (Remember that in yogic terms, these are known as brahmana practices—heating and energizing.) In particular, revisit the practices Lengthening the Inhalation (page 108) and Extending the Pause after Inhalation (page 104) in week 4.

When you're feeling slothful, the last thing you may want to do is jump into a vigorous vinyasa of back bends and handstands. In that case, ease your body awake through supported back bends such as the following familiar heart-opening pose over a bolster—and add a three-part inhalation and a pause after the inhalation to increase the energizing benefits.

PRACTICE 11.50
Gentle Supported Back Bend with Three-Part Inhalation (10 minutes)

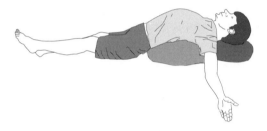

For this practice you need a yoga bolster and a meditation cushion. If you don't have a bolster, you can make one by stacking up three firm, folded yoga blankets or taking a square zabuton (meditation mat) and folding it in a zigzag accordion fold.

Place your bolster crosswise about a third of the way down your mat, with your meditation cushion a few inches behind it. Then lie back over the bolster with it positioned just behind your heart. The very tops of your shoulders will extend slightly over the edge of the bolster. Rest the back of your skull on your meditation cushion and release your arms into the space between the bolster and the cushion, with the backs of the hands resting on the floor. You should feel a delicious opening, not an intense stretch. If this is too much of a back bend for you, lower the height of the support: use two or just one folded blanket instead of a bolster.

Extend the legs or, if you feel any pinching in the lower back, keep the knees bent with the soles of the feet flat on the floor.

Rest in the pose for 3 to 5 minutes, paying close attention to the sensations in your body and breath. Then, after a natural inhalation, let the breath out completely. Inhale to about a third of your lung capacity and pause for just a heartbeat, with no strain. Inhale another third, then pause. Inhale the rest of the way and lightly pause at the top of the inhalation, keeping the throat relaxed and open. Then smoothly and slowly let the breath all the way out.

Repeat this breath cycle 5 to 10 times. Empty out any tension in the neck, throat, jaw, and eyes as you suspend the breath.

Then let the breath return to its natural rhythms. Notice the effects.

Going further. Once you've become comfortable with the three-part inhale, you can heighten its effects with the light application of *bandhas* at the throat and the pelvic floor. Commonly translated as "locks," bandhas are better thought of as guardians of the body's energy gates that channel the flow of prana and heighten its effects. So try this: At the end of your three-part inhale, while suspending the breath at the top, delicately draw up on the pelvic floor in a light Mula Bandha (root lock). At the same time, soften the throat and drop the chin toward the breastbone in Jalandhara Bandha (throat lock). Suspend the breath and engage the bandhas for about 3 counts. Then release. Practice 3 to 5 times. Then let the breath return to its natural rhythms.

PRACTICE 11.51
Alternate-Nostril Breathing (5–15 minutes)

Centuries ago, yogis noticed what modern science has now confirmed—that the inner linings of the left and right nostrils shrink and swell in a rhythmic, synchronized cycle of roughly ninety minutes, so that the breath is usually dominant in one nostril or the other. When you breathe in and out through the right nostril, blood pressure and heart rate increase, along with other signs of sympathetic nervous system dominance—in other words, your body and mind are preparing for action. Breathe in and out the left nostril and they decrease, as your body shifts into parasympathetic mode of relaxation and letting go.

The familiar practice of Alternate-Nostril Breathing is a powerful way to bring the qualities of energy and tranquillity back into balance in your nervous system. It can also be used as an antidote for either sleepiness or restlessness, the next hindrance on our list.

Alternate-Nostril Breathing can be practiced either sitting or lying down. There are many traditional variations on the hand gesture, or mudra, for practicing alternate-nostril breathing. Here we'll use the most simple— just extend the index and middle finger of the right hand while folding down the ring finger and pinky. Touch the extended fingers to the third eye (the area just between and slightly above your eyebrows). Exhale through both nostrils. Then cover your right nostril with the right thumb while inhaling and exhaling through the left nostril.

Breathe several rounds through the left nostril. Notice any prickling as the breath moves through the sinus cavity, the slight dryness as it passes down into the throat. With every inhalation through the left nostril, feel the whole left side of your body light up: the left side of the skull and face, left torso and arm, left side of the pelvis, left leg. Every inhalation awakens sensitivity in the left side of your body; every exhalation drains away unconscious gripping.

After 5 to 10 complete cycles, at the top of your inhalation through the left nostril, close off the left nostril with the right ring finger. Lift the right thumb from the right nostril and exhale on the right side. Now let the whole right side of your body light up as the breath flows in and out the right nostril.

After 5 to 10 cycles on this side, begin to alternate the inhale and exhale. After you inhale on the right, exhale on the left. Then inhale on the left and exhale on the right. As you switch from one side to the other, feel your attention flow with your breath back and forth across the midline of your body.

Practice 5 to 10 full rounds, alternating with every breath. After your final inhalation on the right, lower your hand and continue the practice with your awareness alone. Without the support of your hand, invite your breath to flow more fully in one nostril, then the other, following the same pattern you have been practicing with the help of the fingers. Bathe in your attention first on one side of the body, then on the other.

After your last inhalation on the right, exhale through both nostrils and return to your natural breath. Notice any effects of the practice.

PRACTICE 11.52
Breath of Joy (3 minutes)

This simple standing breath practice makes a good energy-boosting break, as well as providing a way to heat up the body and wake up the mind in preparation for a longer practice.

Begin in Standing Meditation (page 145) tuning in to the natural rhythms of the breath. Now begin a vigorous, sniffing three-part inhalation, accompanied by a swinging upward of the arms, almost as if you were conducting an orchestra: Inhale as the arms rise in front of you to shoulder height, then briefly pause; continue the inhale as the arms swoop out to the sides level with the shoulders, and pause again; then swing the arms toward each other and all the way overhead as you complete the last inhaling sniff. Then exhale through the mouth with a loud, vigorous *ha!* as you lower the arms.

Repeat 5 to 10 times, then release back to Standing Meditation. Take some time to notice the effects on the mind and heart.

Opportunity 4: Restlessness

You know that jittery, anxious feeling that whatever you are doing, you really should be doing something else instead? In our multitasking world, this restlessness is a chronic condition—we're constantly checking our e-mail while talking on the phone to one person and texting another.

Sometimes compulsive multitasking is just a way of masking a free-floating anxiety that may be driving our busyness. When we're forced to slow down for even a short while—such as in the enforced stillness of a meditation retreat—this anxiety can bubble up. And just sitting and observing it can often make it worse, like being locked in an echo chamber with someone reading your to-do list over a loudspeaker.

On one retreat where I taught, one of the yogis became so anxious from the seated meditation that she couldn't sleep at night. She barricaded the door to her room with her chair—piled high with her suitcase and clothes—so no one could break in. For her, sitting in stillness quickly became unbearable. She needed a more active and engaging breath-and-movement practice—like the ones I offer below—that would give her restless brain something to do while at the same time soothing her nervous system so she could move more deeply into stillness.

In our culture most of us are chronically stuck with the accelerator of the sympathetic nervous system pressed down—if we were a car, there would be a worldwide factory recall. Our nervous systems are constantly on red alert, preparing to fight off saber-toothed e-mails. Our muscles are tensed to flee from woolly mammoth–sized conference calls. Our amygdala—the almond-shaped node deep in our reptilian brain that monitors danger—goes into overdrive, instructing our nervous system to scan the horizon, looking for what's about to go wrong.

Whether your restlessness manifests as a mind seething with plans that can't be switched off, insomnia, preperformance jitters, or just low-grade background anxiety, yoga postures and breath practices can be a useful tool. Yoga enables us to shift deliberately from our culture's dominant mode of sympathetic hypervigilance into the deep stillness of parasympathetic dominance. It lowers levels of the stress hormone cortisol. And it increases levels in the brain of an important neurotransmitter called gamma-aminobutyric acid, or GABA, which slows down the firing of neurons, promoting muscular relaxation and reducing anxiety.

Responses

As you recall from week 4, pranayama practices that lengthen and emphasize the exhalation and extend the pause afterward are especially powerful tools for soothing a restless mind. So reacquaint yourself with Lengthening the Exhalation (page 108) and Extending the Pause after Exhalation (page 102).

If you're feeling restless or agitated, long-held forward bends, supported inversions, and shoulder stands are all poses that particularly aid in the shift from the sympathetic to the parasympathetic nervous system. That said, it's important to meet yourself where you are; trying to drop immediately into a slow practice of long holds may just exacerbate your agitation. So if you have a hard time being still, do a more dynamic yoga practice but emphasize the exhalations and the holds after exhalations during your flow (see practice 11.56, Moving on the Hold after Exhalation). The goal isn't to wear yourself out through sweaty vinyasa so you're too tired to be anxious. While that may be effective in the short term, it won't address the underlying patterns of tension and anxiety, which will reemerge as soon as you're rested again. The goal is to move the nervous system skillfully into a state of more grounded balance.

PRACTICE 11.53
Exhaling into Peace (5 minutes)

Adding imagery to your pranayama practice can heighten its power.

In a comfortable reclining or sitting position, connect with the exhalation and the pause after the exhalation. Drop into the pause after the exhalation, and in that pause, summon an image that gives you a deep sense of peace and well-being. Perhaps you see yourself in a favorite spot in nature that always soothes your heart. Or imagine yourself with a beloved grandmother. If no image comes, just say a word to yourself: *Peace.* Or *Ease.* Or *Joy.* Let yourself relax into the feeling that the image or word evokes as you continue to suspend the breath for just a few heartbeats.

Then let the inhale wash back in like a wave over the sand. As the inhale washes through you, be filled with the feeling of peace and ease that the image evoked in you.

Repeat this breath cycle 5 to 15 times. Then let your breath return to normal. Invite the feelings of ease and well-being to continue to expand through your whole being as you rest in the natural breath.

PRACTICE 11.54
Three-Part Exhalation (10 minutes)

This practice heightens even further the soothing effect of focusing on the exhalation.

As always, begin your breath practice by getting familiar with your breath just as it is. When you are restless, your breath may be shallow, tense, and uneven. Can you be okay with that?

After a normal inhalation, exhale a third of the way, as if pouring a third of the water out of a glass. Pause for just a heartbeat, then exhale another third. Pause again, then exhale all the way out. Pause for a heartbeat or so at the bottom of your exhalation, making sure that you have let out all the breath. Gather the lower belly back. Then release the lower belly and allow the inhalation to flow in naturally, without pulling at it. You may find that the inhalation is slower or fuller than usual, but don't try to create a deep breath deliberately.

Repeat this three-part exhalation for 5 to 10 rounds, then let the breath return to its natural rhythms. Notice the effects.

Try this. Practice the Three-Part Exhalation as described, but add in the visualization practice detailed in practice 11.53: Exhaling into Peace. During the pause after your completed exhalation, invite in an image or word that evokes calm and ease in your being. Drink that feeling in as you inhale. How does this practice enhance the calming effect of the Three-Part Exhalation?

PRACTICE 11.55
Circular Left-Nostril Breathing (3–5 minutes)

This is a variation of Alternate-Nostril Breathing that emphasizes calming over energizing by always inhaling through the left nostril and exhaling through the right. It can be practiced either sitting or lying down.

Just as you did with Alternate-Nostril Breathing, take your right hand and place the first two fingers lightly between and just above the eyebrows. Take a long, smooth inhale and exhale. Then cover the right nostril with your thumb and breathe in through the left nostril. At the top of the inhalation, lift the thumb and cover the left nostril with your ring finger. Breathe out through the right nostril.

Once again, cover the right nostril and breathe in through the left; then cover the left and breathe out through the right. Continue like this—always breathing in through the left nostril and breathing out through the right. Invite the breath to be slow, deep, and even.

As you inhale through the left nostril, sense the left side of your body brightening. As you exhale through the right, sense the right side relaxing.

After 10 rounds, lower your hand and continue the pattern for 5 to 10 more rounds, using just the power of your focused attention to guide the breath. Then return to a natural breath and notice the effects of the practice.

PRACTICE 11.56
Moving on the Hold after Exhalation (5 minutes)

This is a way to emphasize the grounding effect of exhalation during your asana practice.

Get onto all fours and warm up by flowing through a few rounds of Cat-Cow—exhale as you draw the belly back and round the spine, inhale as you arch the spine (page 61). Then remain on all fours with the spine in neutral and exhale completely, gathering the lower belly back at the bottom of the exhalation. While still holding out the breath, press back into Downward Dog—moving on the empty pause. Notice how the lower belly naturally engages and sucks back even farther as you do so. This creates a natural *uddiyana bandha*—a classic yogic technique for harnessing and focusing the energy in that part of the body.

Inhale and exhale in Downward Dog for a couple of breaths. Then exhale as you lower your knees back down to your mat. Inhale on all fours. Exhale fully. Moving on the empty pause—holding the breath out—press back into Downward Dog. Then inhale and exhale naturally in the pose.

Repeat this cycle a few more times, always moving on the empty pause. Notice how moving on empty extends the pause after exhalation. After a few rounds of this, notice the effect on your breath, body, and mind.

Going further. This is a very soothing and grounding technique to use in the midst of a flowing practice. Once you've gotten comfortable with it in this simple sequence, you can use it throughout your asana flow. Whenever you would normally have moved on an exhalation—say, from standing into a forward bend—instead move on the pause *after* the exhalation. What do you notice?

Opportunity 5: Doubt

On the second day of a meditation retreat, I met a yogi wheeling her suitcase to the parking lot. "I can't believe I came here when I could have gone to a spa in Napa," she snapped.

On the meditative path, doubt manifests as persistent questions that undermine our ability to carry on: *Why am I doing this? Is this the right path for me? Who are these idiots anyway?* Sometimes doubt arises when you've hit a plateau—you made such great strides as you were starting out, but now you can't see any progress. Maybe a practice that used to serve you well no longer works for you. Or maybe you've become disillusioned because a teacher whose method you put your faith in has behaved in unethical ways. You might value the practice but doubt your own abilities: *Other people can meditate, but I can't.*

Some measure of doubt is an essential element of the spiritual path—so that you aren't taking your practice on blind faith but are testing it in the crucible of your intelligent investigation. A Zen proverb says that to progress on the path, a student must have great faith, great doubt, and great determination. But too much doubt can be paralyzing—so much so that you never pick up the stick of practice to begin with. It can undermine your enthusiasm for your efforts, making it impossible for you to tackle with determination any of the other hindrances. Why work hard to travel a path you're not sure leads to the right place—especially when you also doubt your own abilities and the encouraging words of others?

Responses

The classic antidote to doubt is faith—not a blind belief in rote principles but a willingness to trust and open to what's actually happening
and see for yourself what is true. If doubt regularly hits at the start of
your practice session, tell yourself that you'll reevaluate your practice
after you've finished for that day, but you won't bail out beforehand.

Then use your practice as a laboratory to test which tools from the
vast yogic tool kit work for you now. Reflect on your highest aspiration
for your life and seek out the practices that best support that vision.
Remind yourself of the teachings that have most inspired and helped
you. Remember, your practice is alive, and life constantly evolves. So
rather than offering you a specific doubt-busting practice, I suggest the
following contemplative meditation.

PRACTICE 11.57
Contemplative Meditation (10 minutes)

---

*Contemplative meditation is a technique for exploring a question not with
your conceptual mind but from the depths of meditative stillness.*

Sit or lie in a comfortable meditative position. Close your eyes and
spend several minutes calming and centering through whatever meditative technique you've explored in this program that works most effectively for you.

Then ask yourself a question, as if dropping it like a pebble into the
clear, still water of your mind: *What practice is right for me right in this
moment?*

Don't chew on this question with your intellect. Just let it settle to
the bottom of your inner pool and rest there. After a minute or so, ask
it again—and again let it drop.

Repeat this several more times. Then sit still and wait for an answer to arise in the form of an image, a word or phrase, or simply an
impulse. It's fine if it's something very simple—in fact, it's probably
better that it is. *I need to do a five-minute Shoulder Stand. I need to dance. I
need to hike to the ocean. I need to grab my journal and write down my*

dreams. All that matters is that when it bubbles up, your body knows that it's right—just for right now.

Then follow that impulse. Don't worry if it seems absurd: just grab your jacket and head to the hills that are calling you. Pull out your dusty box of watercolors and begin to paint. Catch on to your intuition like the end of a golden thread and follow it through the labyrinth of doubt and back to the heart of your own aliveness.

In Your Daily Life This Week

As you go through your day, notice what tends to sweep you away from your connection with the present, moment by moment. If you catch yourself adrift in a sea of thoughts or emotions, take the time to investigate: Is one of the Five Hindrances whipping up the waves? If you find a particular hindrance cropping up again and again, focus on it in your formal practice.

RESOURCES

Much of what I know about working with hindrances through yoga came from my dear friend and colleague Janice Gates; see her somatic yoga therapy training at www.janicegates.com. I also recommend Amy Weintraub's excellent *Yoga Skills for Therapists*. G. I. Fronsdale's book *Unhindered: A Mindful Path through the Five Hindrances* is an excellent guide to the classic Buddhist approach. To highlight joy and well-being in your meditation practice, try James Baraz's book and online course, *Awakening Joy*.

Living Joyfully with Impermanence

ON A GUSTY, brilliant spring morning when Skye was seven years old, we stepped out our front door into a wind-tossed shower of falling plum blossoms. Wrens bustled and gossiped in the wine-red leaves of the Japanese maple that arches over our gate.

"What an amazing day!" I said, slinging an arm around his shoulder and pulling him close.

"It *is* amazing!" he agreed. He paused, then added cheerfully, "Of course, the sun could already have exploded and we wouldn't even know it for another eight minutes."

That just about sums up the precarious, astonishing reality that we live in. (For those of you who aren't up on your second-grade science, it takes about eight minutes for the light from the sun to reach the earth.) Our lives are almost unbearably gorgeous—and they could end at any moment. Everything and everyone that we love will eventually blow away like fog on a windy beach.

I once read a collection of ordinary people's six-word memoirs—all solicited online—entitled "Not Quite What I Was Planning" (this title is one person's memoir in its entirety). You get some interesting narratives when you sum up a life in six words: "After Harvard, had baby with crackhead." "Found true love, married someone else." But my favorite is this one, which reads like a universal epitaph: "Started small, grew, peaked, shrunk, vanished."

So how do we live in harmony with so much beauty and so much loss—hummingbirds flitting through pineapple sage, children bleeding to death in bombed cities? How do we wake up to the preciousness of our fleeting lives without contracting, numbing out, or hanging on so tight to the things and people we love that our fingertips bleed?

On meditation retreats in the vipassana tradition, we often chant an ancient Pali teaching that's been recited by monks and nuns every day since the time of the Buddha. Its English translation goes: *All things are impermanent. They arise and they pass away. To live in harmony with this truth brings great happiness.*

What a remarkable thing to say! We don't chant: *All things are impermanent, they arise and they pass away—it really sucks, but you better get used to it.* Our practice tells us that we can live in harmony with even the most wrenching forms of impermanence—broken necks, shattered dreams, burning forests, dying friends—while keeping our hearts tender and our actions kind. It tells us that learning the art of living wisely in an unstable world—without denying our human griefs and longings—brings a profound and unshakable joy. And when you settle yourself deep inside your ever-changing body temple of breath and bone, you can feel that joy bubbling up.

This final week of our twelve-week program, we'll turn our attention to exploring—in and through our mindful yoga practice—what the Buddha called the "three characteristics" that are true of our lives in this world: the fact that things are always changing (*anicca*, or impermanence); the stress that arises when we cling to these changing things and circumstances as the source of our happiness (*dukkha*, or suffering); and the freedom that is possible when we open to the reality that we are not permanent, separate entities but are inextricably interconnected with everything and everyone (*anatta*, or no separate self).

In a sense, the ability to know these fundamental truths—not as concepts but as lived understanding—is what this whole course has been building. Over the weeks of this program, you've developed the art of connecting, in sensuous, moment-to-moment presence, with your body, breath, heart, and mind. And along the way you've come to know from the inside out how body sensations, breath, emotions, and thoughts all arise and pass away within your awareness—that none of these things are who you truly are.

Now you'll look directly at the nature of this ever-changing flow—

putting your relationship with it in the foreground of your attention. Through your mindful yoga practice, you'll study how to live in freedom in relationship with the way the world actually is.

THE TRUTH OF IMPERMANENCE

Skye likes to tell a joke about two cows grazing in a field: "Have you heard about that mad cow disease?" one of them asks the other. The other replies, "What do I care about that? I'm a helicopter!"

That's how most of us relate to the open secret of impermanence. Intellectually, we know it's true—but secretly we're convinced that it really doesn't apply to us. When Arjuna asks Krishna in the Bhagavad Gita what the greatest marvel on earth is, Krishna responds, "That all around, human beings see people dying, but you do not believe it will happen to you."

A visceral knowledge of impermanence is one of the most important gifts that a body-based contemplative practice gives us—by pointing our attention toward the ever-changing nature of what we long to perceive as solid.

In his teachings on mindfulness of the body, the Buddha instructs practitioners to go into the forest, sit cross-legged under a tree, and pay attention to different aspects of embodied experience: sensing the breath and the physical posture, feeling into the components and elemental energies that make up the body, imagining it as a corpse in various stages of decay. For each contemplation, the instruction is this: "The monk or nun abides contemplating the nature of arising in the body, or he abides contemplating the nature of passing away in the body, or she abides contemplating the nature of both arising and passing away in the body."

When I was at Plum Village, we used to sit under a tree—in front of the old stone meditation hall that used to be a farm stable—and recite the Five Remembrances that Buddhist monks and nuns have recited daily since the time of the Buddha:

I am of the nature to grow old. There is no way to escape growing old.

I am of the nature to have ill health. There is no way to escape ill health.

I am of the nature to die. There is no way to escape death.

All that is dear to me and everyone I love is of the nature to change.

There is no way to escape being separated from them.

Really, it's amazing that we manage to forget these remembrances as much as we do—because if you're paying attention at all, it's pretty hard to avoid the fact that bodies change.

Recently I went to a class at a yoga studio where they had wall-to-wall mirrors, something I haven't faced for years in my yoga practice, since I practice mainly at home. I lifted up into a headstand and looked face-to-face at my upside-down image with astonishment: *Huh! I don't recall that when I used to do Headstand, my entire face collapsed into a pile on my forehead!*

Pay attention in your yoga practice, and your body's changes will stare right at you, day by day and year by year—as you get stronger or weaker, get sick or heal, get pregnant, get injured, and gradually get old. Yoga can help shape the way your body changes over time—but it can't drive away forever the yipping coyotes of sickness, old age, and death. Over the years, the bodies of many of my longtime yoga friends have broken down: strokes, surgeries, cancer, chronic anxiety, or depression. They've had to change the way they practiced to meet their bodies' changing needs—substituting restorative postures for handstands, learning to sense the subtle fluctuations of sensation in the spine rather than mastering a picture-perfect back bend—and along the way, they've acquired ever-deepening insights into the nature and purpose of practice itself.

And the impermanence of our bodies doesn't just reveal itself over long periods of time. Each breath arises and disappears, as shape-shifting as a cloud. Body sensations sparkle and sing and flash in and out. An ache turns into a tingle turns into a glow, then melts away. You feel your way into a hip or a shoulder that seems to be solid—and it begins to swirl like water, drift like mist.

Three hundred million cells die in your body every minute; three hundred billion more are born every day. Every hour you shed six hundred thousand particles of skin. You manufacture a new stomach lining every three to four days. Nerve impulses to and from your brain are traveling at a speed of 170 miles per hour.

Even at your stillest, most meditative moments, you are in constant motion. And your yoga asana practice gives you a chance to experience yourself directly as the ever-changing flow that you are.

THE TRUTH OF SUFFERING

So once you start to get a visceral feel for this truth of impermanence, what do you do?

Well, here's one approach you can try: hold on tight, as hard as you can, for as long as you can.

This is the approach that's generally recommended by our culture, especially when it comes to our bodies. We're constantly scrambling to find the right combination to the immortality safe: Are eggs good or bad this week? Should I be feasting on red wine and chocolate or wheatgrass juice and quinoa? Is brown rice macrobiotic manna or a high-glycemic carbo-bomb?

And why just stop with preserving your body? A website called LivesOn, dedicated to "your social afterlife," ensures that your Twitter feed remains active after you are dead. Their slogan: "When your heart stops beating, you'll keep tweeting."

If we're not careful, the pursuit of permanence can creep into our yoga practice as well. It's a belief that's been part of the hatha yoga mythology since the very beginning: that by dint of your diligent practice, you can create a "diamond body" that's impervious to death. Certainly yoga asana practice can work wonders in terms of keeping our bodies healthy and fit into old age. (Although it's also possible, of course, for yoga practice to injure them. An orthopedic surgeon once told me, "Every time I hear that someone has started doing yoga, I think *Great! Another payment on my Lexus.*"). But if we hang on to the body's eternal youth as the reason for our practice and a necessary element for our happiness, we are setting ourselves up for severe disappointment. Because the truth of impermanence leads us straight to the second of the three characteristics of existence—the fact that if we pin our happiness on things that are impermanent, we're going to have a hard time.

The Pali word for this truth is *dukkha*—it's often translated as "suffering," but that's not quite accurate. The word *dukkha* derives from the word for a dirty axle hole—the term was originally used to describe what happened when the axle hole of an oxcart got packed with dirt so the wheel couldn't turn properly. Life, the Buddha is telling us, can be a bumpy ride.

In a world where everything is changing, you're bound to experience this jarring and jolting to varying degrees again and again. There's the physical stress of your body's getting sick, injured, or just uncomfortable—running the gamut from the discomfort of sitting on a hard bench at a boring lecture to the agony of brain cancer. And then there is emotional struggle, from small irritations to devastating heartbreak: You're hungry and you just burned your dinner. The person you love is an addict. Polar bears are drowning as glaciers melt into the sea. Your best friend's car skidded on black ice and went over a cliff.

As yoga practitioners, sometimes we feel that we're supposed to be immune to physical and emotional disaster. I've known yoga teachers who were too embarrassed to tell their students they were sick or injured or had to have surgery: How could their students have faith in the practice if it didn't protect the teacher's body from breaking down? Back in the early nineties, I started to research an article for *Yoga Journal* by interviewing well-known senior yoga teachers about how their bodies and their practice had changed as they got older. I had to abandon the article because most of them didn't want to be included in an article about getting older and didn't want to admit publicly that their practice had changed in any way, lest it frighten off their younger clientele.

And admitting to emotional challenges can be even more difficult. I was embarrassed to tell my meditation teachers I was getting a divorce just a couple of years after I'd gotten married—how could this be happening to a good Buddhist like me, especially after all of those books I'd bought on relationship as a spiritual practice? When a close friend of mine struggled with depression and anxiety, she felt like a failure as a yoga teacher.

So just turning toward and acknowledging the bumpiness of life can be a huge relief. These pains and heartbreaks aren't our personal failure—they don't mean that something has gone terribly wrong. They are just the way life in an ever-changing world sometimes is.

Life shimmers with beauty and magic, and our practice helps us connect with this luminous mystery again and again. But acknowledging the universality of suffering means that we don't have to push away all the dark, scary, and painful parts of our bodies, our hearts, and our lives. We can honor the whole situation, even when it hurts. And that kind of opening brings both relief and a kind of dignity.

We can also see the way we are making the situation worse by obsessively clinging to what can't be kept forever. It's natural to cherish and care for people and things and experiences we love. Who wants to say good-bye forever to a beloved sister's laughter, the scudding of cirrus clouds across a desert sky? It's life affirming to enjoy a sweet tangerine, a salty sea wind, the caress of a hand on skin; to do everything we can to heal a sick friend, to mend a torn muscle, to plant trees in a deforested river valley.

But when that appreciation and care hardens into obsessive craving—*I've got to make this go my way or I can't be happy!*—we're doomed. Because ultimately, we're going to have to let go of it all. Even in the most enchanted life, our children grow up and the people we love grow old—and we ourselves catapult triumphantly across the finish line past the cheering crowd and into the grave.

So how can your yoga asana practice help you live skillfully with life's inevitable losses?

First of all, your asana practice can help you learn to open to and feel what the vipassana teacher Phillip Moffitt calls the "ouch" of your hard times—to enter into your struggles as a felt sensation in the body without flinching away. In week 8 you practiced getting intimate with unpleasant sensations as well as pleasant ones: *An aching hip feels like this. A hurt shoulder feels like that.* Now you can use that capacity—both on your yoga mat and in your life—to recognize when a painful moment is arising. *I'm so disappointed I didn't get that job. I'm so sad that my grandmother broke her hip.* You can feel the way the sorrow tightens into a lump in your throat or pressure in your chest. Just naming the painful emotion can create a little spaciousness around it. You don't deny or belittle your pain or try to minimize its significance. Nor do you dump its paint bucket all over your life: *Life is full of suffering, so I'll never be happy.* You just recognize that this moment of struggle is a normal part of human life.

Second, asana can be a laboratory for studying how you respond to those moments. When your yoga poses get uncomfortable, do you hastily move on to more pleasurable ones? Do you avoid the poses you aren't good at so you don't feel challenged or embarrassed? Do you push into pain further and injure yourself? Do you numb out? Do you tell yourself that your pain is not important? Whatever strategies you're using in your yoga practice are likely to be at play in your life as well.

You can use your asana practice to look at the ways you create more suffering for yourself by grasping: for more-advanced poses, for more-exotic sensations, for a different body from the one you actually have in the moment—perhaps the body you had ten years ago or the body the person on the next mat has right now. You can learn to track the way that clinging manifests in your body: tension behind the eyes, a clenched jaw, held breath, a flutter of anxiety under your collarbone.

And finally, you can learn to soften that obsessive gripping directly, in your body. This doesn't mean that you stop working toward strength, openness, and energy. You just melt the anxious contraction that may be accompanying and even fueling your movement toward well-being.

This physical softening around your clinging is a potent skill to carry into your life. Because letting go of craving doesn't mean eradicating your desires: for love, for peace, for well-being, for peppermint ice cream, for good education for all children, for an end to gun violence, for diving into a clear mountain lake. It just means loosening the tentacles that you have wrapped around what you want, giving you more freedom to enjoy what you have and not pine for what you don't have.

Every thought leaves a trace in the body. We hang on tight to our yearnings and dreams with the napes of our necks, the roofs of our mouths, the roots of our tongues: *I won't breathe again until I get what I want. It hurts too much to lose what I love, so I will harden my body from the arches of my feet to the pelvic floor to the bones of my skull so I don't feel the heartbreak.*

But through our practice, we find that it is by softening into our pain that we bear it. It is by releasing our clutch on *I want, I need, I must have, I've got to be* that we can open to a deeper kind of joy.

We mourn our losses with all the depth and tenderness of our human hearts. But we don't add to that grief the terrible pain of railing against the way things are, as if life had broken a contract with us that everything we want would be ours forever.

THE TRUTH OF NO SEPARATE SELF

And here's some good news: as we release our stranglehold on the things that we want and become more and more at ease in the dance of impermanence, the third of the three characteristics naturally begins to flower in our understanding. Nothing remains the same for even an instant—even subatomic particles are constantly dancing. So nothing has a solid, separate self—even what you think of as "me." This doesn't just mean that "I exist for a while as a solid entity, but eventually I, too, will pass away." It means that this "I" that seems so solid and separate is just an illusion. It doesn't have an unchanging core. And because of that, it is completely interconnected with everything else. As Thich Nhat Hanh says, "We inter-are."

Feel into your body and you know this directly. Your body sings you the whole story: You are made of the yogurt you had for breakfast and the grass eaten by the cows who made that milk and the rain that fell on their pastures and the sun's heat and light. You are made of mountain streams and your mother's passion for your father's touch and particles born at the dawn of the universe. I hear my grandmother's voice echo in the throats of her great-great-grandchildren. When my son is asleep, his mouth looks just like his dad's—and like the pictures of the grandfather who died before he was born.

As you pay attention to the landscape of your thoughts, you've probably noticed that your inner narrative constantly changes, tossing up shifting, imaginary versions of the Fascinating Story of You. This understanding can help you relax the painful fixation on *I-me-mine* that drives so much of what people do. Your body-mind arises out of a set of what the Buddha called "causes and conditions": elements coming together for a short while to make something you think of as "me" and then dispersing and recombining again. Your bones will be reborn as seawater and caterpillars. A smile you gave a lonely stranger on a street corner may ripple around the world for a thousand years.

Because of this interconnectedness, impermanence is actually good news. "Thanks to impermanence, everything is possible," said Thich Nhat Hanh in an interview in the *Shambhala Sun*. "Life itself is possible. If a grain of corn is not impermanent, it can never be transformed into a stalk of corn. If the stalk were not impermanent, it could never provide us with the ear of corn we eat. If your daughter is not impermanent, she cannot grow up to become a woman. Then your grandchildren would never manifest. So instead of complaining about impermanence, we should say, 'Warm welcome and long live impermanence.'"

These are not intellectual understandings. They are realizations that penetrate you over and over again, every day, in your cells, in your bones, in your breath.

In your asana practice, you can notice how every part of your body is connected to and is affected by every other part. Grip your jaw and your pelvic floor tightens. Stand on your head and your mood gets brighter. Does your arm begin at your shoulder joint? Or are its roots deep in your heart, in your belly? Can your foot walk without your ankle, knee, and hip?

As you move and breathe on your mat, you can contemplate all of the elements—outside what you think of as "you"—without which your body and your yoga practice could not exist. Could you do pranayama without oxygen? If not, then the arboreal forests of Canada are part of your wider body—as are the rains that watered them and the sea winds that brought the clouds and the sun that shone on the chlorophyll in their leaves. Your bones could not support your weight if it weren't for calcium—pulled from the earth by the roots of kale and pasture grass, forged in the belly of stars. The building blocks of the architecture of your eyes and ears and nose were developed by prehistoric sea creatures. You share more than 90 percent of your DNA with a mouse, and more than 50 percent with a banana.

When you learn to see the world with these eyes, you'll navigate the bumpy roads of impermanence with more ease. You'll be able to see the grandmother you lost in your niece's quick fingers as they move across the piano keys. You'll be able to feel how your love for a friend who died long ago continues to nourish your heart as you care for your friends who are still alive. In the bright light of impermanence and no separate self, you'll remember to cherish the people you love, the redwoods you walk under, the swelling green tomatoes in your garden. Because you know that impermanence doesn't mean that the world won't be here tomorrow. It will be here—but different. And the way you care for it shapes the way it—and you—will change.

WEEK 12 PRACTICES

This week's practices are not specific techniques but targeted contemplations that you can explore within any pose or sequence of poses. Each one also contains instructions for related explorations in your seated meditation and in your daily life.

On days 1 and 2, practice Knowing Your Changing Body; days 3 and 4, Getting Comfortable with Discomfort; days 5 and 6, Knowing No Separate Self. The final day, choose whichever exploration seemed richest and go further with it.

PRACTICE 12.58
Knowing Your Changing Body (30–60 minutes)

This contemplation of impermanence can be done in any sequence of yoga poses: You can choose a sequence you're familiar with and flow through it, map out a new one in advance, or improvise your practice pose by pose and let it surprise you. If you're not sure what to do, use the same sequence that you used to explore emotions in week 9 (Asana Sequence for Tracking Emotions, page 197).

Begin your practice with Checking In with Body, Heart, and Mind (5.28 on page 130). Find out what's true on this day in your body, your heart, and your mind. At the end of your meditation, jot down a few words in your journal that describe each level of your being. *Body: bloated, sore knee. Heart: anxious. Mind: repeatedly going over personal budget.*

Then set a timer to chime throughout your asana practice at 10-minute intervals. Each time it chimes, perform another brief check-in and jot the words down again.

As you're practicing, notice the qualities of change in your practice itself—how one pose dissolves fluidly into the next. Warrior gives way to Triangle; Downward Dog flows to Upward Dog. Sometimes this transformation happens rapidly, in a nonstop vinyasa; sometimes the changes are more slow and deliberate as you linger over particular stages of your journey. But nothing is ever static.

Deliberately include some time in your practice where these changes are rapid—where you move from pose to pose without holding anything for longer than 5 breaths. How do you relate to the constant changes? Do you find yourself holding on to favorite poses and wishing you could stay? Or are you constantly leaning into the next exciting change without fully resting in the pose you are in? Can you fully inhabit each shape, even knowing that it is going to change very soon? Are you someone who thrives on constant change and gets bored when things seem static? Or does change make you anxious?

Also include some time to practice long, slow holds—holding each pose for at least 5 minutes before moving on to the next. Use each pose as a meditation, tuning in to some aspect of your experience— body sensations, breath—and staying with it steadily. Notice the changing nature of what superficially appears to be static. Sense the ebb and flow of the breath, the beating of your heart, the changing temperature of your skin. Enter into the living chamber of a joint or an organ and feel what you thought was solid dissolve into a whirling sea of sensations. Feel the tides of emotions, the flicker of thoughts.

At the close of your practice, look back over your notes. What changed in your body, heart, and mind? What stayed the same?

In your seated meditation. If your mind drifts, don't berate yourself as you return to your anchor. Instead, take it as just another manifestation of how everything changes. Your attention focuses for a while, then disperses. Your heart is a calm sea; then the wind starts to whip up the whitecaps. This is normal. It's not your personal flaw.

In your life. Off the mat and the cushion, continue to notice how everything changes and how you relate to that fact. You bundle up for a hike in the fog; then the sun rolls in and you peel off the layers. Your baby is cranky, then giggling, then asleep. You're in a great mood, then you read your e-mail—and suddenly you're stressed, anxious, and irritable. You give away a pile of clothes that used to fit. You read your old journals: what happened to the person who wrote them, who was so wound up about crises and goals you can't even remember anymore?

PRACTICE 12.59
Getting Comfortable with Discomfort (30–60 minutes)

In this contemplation you'll use your asana practice as a laboratory for exploring your relationship with life's inevitable struggles—in particular, the uncomfortable sensations and emotions that arise in the course of your practice.

Like the previous practice, this one can be done in any style or sequence of poses. If you want to make sure you have plenty of material to work with, include a lot of those poses you hate and normally try to avoid—you know what they are. Or go back and revisit the Hard Times practice from week 8 (page 184).

Study how you respond to the moments of struggle that arise. Do you wallow in them? Avoid them? Deny them? Think about something else? Attempt to make them disappear? Instead, see if you can let yourself feel the sting of them without flinching away. Develop your capacity to know that this is just a difficult moment—and that it is okay. This doesn't mean that you push yourself too hard or stay in injurious postures. It just means that you leave enough space around your discomfort that you can consciously respond to it rather than reflexively reacting.

Observe, too, if you find yourself straining to hang on to or amplify pleasant sensations, striving for more dramatic or "advanced" postures, or pushing yourself further than your body is ready for. Are there ways that you actually create suffering for yourself through your yoga practice—rather than alleviating it—by comparing yourself to an imaginary ideal? If you're in a yoga class, are you comparing your body, your practice, your outfits, and your overall spiritual worthiness to those of the people around you?

All of these are forms of clinging that take you out of what's actually happening. Notice how painful that grasping is. Where does it live in your body? Invite that tight belly to release, that tense tongue to rest, that gripped jaw to unhinge, that caught breath to flow out. Experience the ease that comes when you soften your resistance to the truth of how things are in the moment—even if the moment itself continues to be painful or challenging.

In your seated meditation. Continue to notice how you relate to the arising of difficult moments—physical pain, emotional storms, dissatisfaction with your own wandering mind. Can you open your heart to receive it all without trying to fix it or push it away? Can you rest in a space that is larger than any of the struggles that might arise within it?

In your life. How do you meet the different forms of minor and major struggle that arise in the course of the day? The physical pains or discomfort? The emotional challenges, big and small? Notice the human tendency to try to arrange and control circumstances so that you never have to experience a moment of dissatisfaction. How is this working for you? See if you can tell the difference—as a felt sense in your body—between demanding that things be other than they are and skillfully working to create well-being for yourself and others.

PRACTICE 12.60
Knowing No Separate Self (20–40 minutes)

One powerful practice for contemplating your interconnectedness with all of life is the classic Buddhist meditation on the four elemental energies of earth, air, water, and fire that manifest in the physical body. One of the fundamental tools for mindfulness of the body, meditating on the four elements can connect you directly to the understanding that you are not separate. In this variation of that traditional contemplation, you'll feel into these four elemental energies as you move through your asana practice.

Like the previous two practices, this contemplation can be done in any asana sequence. It's particularly suited to the kind of free-form exploration we did in week 2. If you need a refresher, return to The Journey of Downward Dog (page 62). Or feel free to let go of formal asanas entirely and release into spontaneous movement.

To aid in this exploration, set a timer to ring every 5 to 10 minutes.

1: Earth. Begin in stillness—standing, sitting, or lying down. Open to the solidity of the earth beneath you. Then sense the energy of the earth in your body, expressing as the qualities of solidity, density, and firmness. Tune in to the weight and heft of your bones. Include in your attention all the other hard parts of your body, such as teeth and fingernails.

As you begin to move into your asana practice, imagine that you can move from your bones—whatever that means for you. Root down into the earth through whatever part of your body is touching it and feel the structure of your skeleton shifting from pose to pose, like a piece of the earth itself in motion. Know that your bones are built of the same minerals as rocky cliffs, fertile meadows, desert sands. Remember that one day they will return to be part of them again. As you move through your postures, ask yourself: *Do these bones belong to me? Are they who I am?*

2: Air. Now, as you continue to practice, shift the focus of your attention from your bones to your breath. Let your body begin to float on as if your breath were blowing through you like the same wild wind that blows through the treetops and over the mountains. Know that you are breathing in the out breath of trees. Remember that every molecule of air you inhale has passed through the bodies of countless creatures before you. Do you remember your first breath? When you breathe your last one, will you know it? As you ride on your breath from pose to pose, wonder: Does your breath belong to you? Is it who you are? Or is it just blowing through you for a little while?

3: Water. Now attune to your fluid nature. Let yourself ripple and flow within and around and between your asanas. Sense the liquids in your body—your blood, your sweat, your saliva, the fluids that bathe your spine and your brain. Your body is 90 percent water. Where does the water come from that you've been drinking this week, that now permeates every cell? A reservoir in distant mountains fed by winter snowmelt? A well in your backyard? Your tears are the exact chemical composition of ocean water. When they fall, is it you who are weeping? Or an ancient sea?

4: Fire. By now your body may be heating up. Feel its warmth. If you could blaze like fire, how would you move? Dance like a flame. Move stronger and faster and feel the heat build. Know that if the sun were extinguished, your life would blow out like a snuffed candle. Does the heat of your blood belong to you?

As you wind down your explorations, drop these questions into your heart: Is this the same body you had when you first started doing yoga—whether yesterday, last year, or decades ago? Does it belong to you and follow all of your commands? Is there an unchanging "I" who controls it, separate from all of its changing, growing, and dying parts?

When you have completed the practice, lie down in Savasana— fluid and solid, breathing and warm. Rest in the center of your ever-changing life, knowing that you are not separate from your world.

In your seated meditation. When you catch yourself lost in thought, notice: Did your spinning wheel of thought revolve around the axis of you? Were you the star of the movie your mind was playing? If so, don't judge yourself—it's nothing personal, it's just what human minds do. It isn't even "your" mind, any more than your body is "your" body. So don't get in a war with it, with the "good" you trying to bring the "bad" you under its control. Remember, neither of these imaginary selves is solid or permanent. So relax a little and smile. Then rest in a space that's larger than anyone you imagine yourself to be.

In your life. Notice all the different selves you incarnate in the course of an ordinary day: The yogi or yogini. The student. The lover. The hardworking professional. The failure. The star. The victim. The good meditator. The bad meditator. Pay attention to the stories you tell yourself—and other people—about who you are. Can you see the way you create your sense of a solid self through your repetitive thoughts? See how it feels, in the middle of a sticky situation, to loosen up the straitjacket of your identity just a little bit.

RESOURCES

The best book I know for learning to live joyfully with the inevitable struggles of an ever-changing world is Phillip Moffitt's *Dancing with Life*. It walks you through a practical, step-by-step program that will transform the way you relate to your life's challenges. Virtually everything that Thich Nhat Hanh writes is saturated with his wisdom around impermanence and interdependence. I especially recommend his *No Death, No Fear* and *The Sun My Heart*.

Acknowledgments

When you practice and teach in a tradition that's thousands of years old, there's really no such thing as "original work." The insights and practices in this book are ones I've integrated in the crucible of my own practice over decades of study with dozens of teachers in both the Buddhist and yogic traditions. Whenever they are drawn primarily from a particular teacher or lineage, I've tried to acknowledge that source specifically—I apologize in advance for any influences I may have inadvertently overlooked.

In the yoga tradition, I bow especially to Angela Farmer, for her intuitive, inner-body approach to asana; Donna Farhi, for her sensitive explorations of breath; Kali Ray, for her creative flows; Richard Miller, for his yoga nidra practice; Ganga White, for his willingness to challenge sacred cows; and my dear friends Sarah Powers, for her yogic integration of traditional Chinese medicine and dharma, and Janice Gates, for her energy balancing sequences and celebration of the power of the feminine. I've learned something from every one of the guest teachers in the Mindfulness Yoga Training that I direct at Spirit Rock—who have included Frank Jude Boccio, Chip Hartranft, Tias Little, Jill Satterfield, and Patricia Sullivan—as well as the many other friends and teachers too numerous to name with whom I have rolled out a sticky mat. And Linda Sparrowe—thank you for keeping me laughing!

In the Buddhist tradition, I honor Maezumi Roshi, my first Zen teacher, who had the courage to reveal his human flaws even on camera; Jack Kornfield, my first vipassana teacher, who masterfully integrates Buddha dharma with Western psychotherapy; Debra Chamberlin-Taylor, who grounds me in the sacred feminine and helps me compost life crises into wisdom; Phillip Moffitt, for his ongoing mentorship of my teaching and practice; and Thich Nhat Hanh, whose teachings on joy, impermanence, interconnectedness, and love are the ground of my practice. A big thank you, too, to all the Buddhist teachers at Spirit Rock Meditation Center on whose retreats I have been privileged to lead yoga sessions over many years—especially the ones I've teamed up with again and again, such as Howard Cohn, Mark Coleman, Anna Douglas, and Julie Wester. It has been a true dharma apprenticeship and I am unendingly grateful for what I have learned from them.

Some passages in this book originally appeared in different form in articles in the *Shambhala Sun, Tricycle: The Buddhist Review, Yoga Journal,* and *Yoga International.* Many thanks to the editors of those fine publications for encouraging my writing over more than two decades.

As a qigong master and Zen teacher, Teja Bell has deepened immeasurably my understanding of the energy body and its relationship to embodied dharma. As a beloved partner, he has kept me happy, juicy, and sane while I wrestled this book into existence.

And my son, Skye Hawthorne, continues to remind me every day that life is a joyful adventure.

Index

About the Author

ANNE CUSHMAN is a pioneer in the integration of creative expression, yoga, and Buddhist mindfulness meditation. She is the director of Mindfulness Yoga and Meditation Training at Spirit Rock Meditation Center in northern California, and teaches regular retreats and courses both in person and online. Since graduating from Princeton University with a degree in comparative religion, she has been a passionate explorer of body-based spiritual practices and their incorporation into the chaos and magic of everyday life. She is the author of the novel *Enlightenment for Idiots* and the spiritual India travel guide *From Here to Nirvana*. Her personal essays on contemplative practice in contemporary life have been widely published in the *New York Times*, the *San Francisco Chronicle*, *O The Oprah Magazine*, *Yoga Journal*, *Yoga International*, and the *Shambhala Sun*. She is a former editor at *Yoga Journal* and *Tricycle: The Buddhist Review*. She lives with her son and her life partner in Fairfax, California. www.annecushman.com